GET OVER IT AND GET ON WITH IT

Using The Ten Principles of Entelechy to
Conquer Change and Create Abundance

Jim Madrid
And
Joyce Quick, M.A., M.S.W.

authorHOUSE®

AuthorHouse™
1663 Liberty Drive, Suite 200
Bloomington, IN 47403
www.authorhouse.com
Phone: 1-800-839-8640

First published by AuthorHouse 9/13/2007

ISBN: 978-1-4343-2633-1 (sc)
ISBN: 978-1-4343-2632-4 (hc)

Library of Congress Control Number: 2007933564

Printed in the United States of America
Bloomington, Indiana

This book is printed on acid-free paper.

Dedicated to:

DARCY MADRID
Jamey Madrid
Jeremy Madrid
Chase Madrid
Devynn Madrid
Ethan Madrid

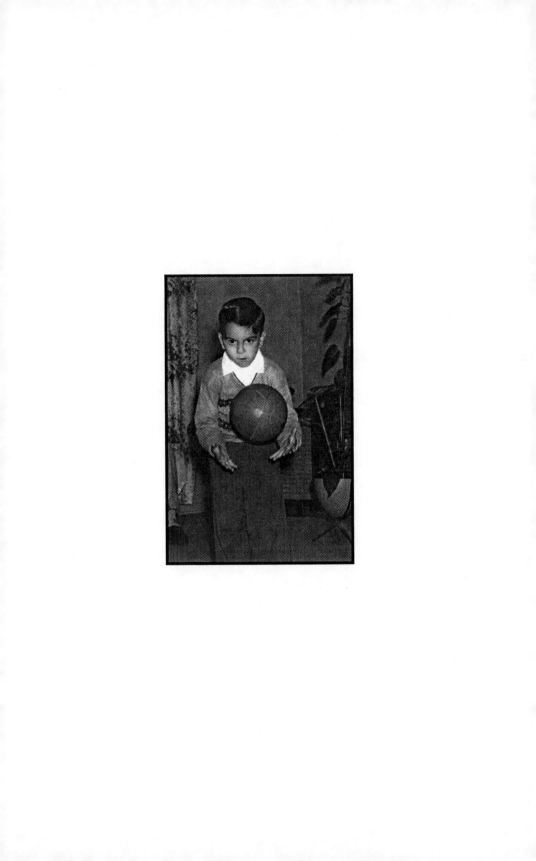

ACKNOWLEDGMENTS

My deepest thanks, gratefulness and love goes to my wife, Darcy. She is my cornerstone for both my personal life and my professional life. She has been pushing me to write this book for years. I love you more today than yesterday.

To my sons, Jamey and Jeremy, for allowing me now to make up all the love and fatherhood that my schooling and training took away from you as I started this journey when you were in high school.

To my son, Chase, for your constant love and dedication to me, whose brilliance is in the design of this book.

To my daughter, Devynn, and my youngest child, Ethan, for understanding when I am on the road away from them; for all their loving voicemails they leave me when I am away.

My family is the reason for a smile on my face and a glow in my heart everyday!

To my friend, confidant, and my co-developer, writer, and editor, Joyce Quick. She has been there through thick and thin. She has kept my feet to the fire and has helped me to stay focused. Your time and effort to this book was immeasurable.

To my friend and mentor, Dr. Nathaniel Branden. Thank you for all the time you have spent with me. Your body of work has not only impacted my life, but my family's and thousands of people who have attended The Ten Principles of Entelechy seminar.

To Father Bob Spitzer, for teaching me what true happiness is all about. I lead my life by Level Three Happiness.

To the gang at Entelechy Training and Development—Jeremy Madrid, Roger Sanford, Jim Hunter, Troy Wyatt, Jaclyn Audeoud at corporate; Richard Rew, Patricia Mendoza in Spain, Bill Cogan and Karen McKenzie in Canada, and John Franich in Seattle. Thanks for all the dedication and great work you do every day.

Steve Rohner, my friend and basketball teammate. Your faith in me has been extraordinary.

A big thanks and appreciation goes to Jim Hagan for his constant support and friendship, and to all of my friends at Fieldstone Mortgage Company.

To Dennis Clements for your trust in me at the very beginning.

To Mr. Bill Heard, thanks for your dedication to constant improvement.

To Roland Arnall for believing in me and giving me a chance.

To Stephen Smythe, thanks for all the words of encouragement and support all these years.

To Billy Cox, for "being in the game."

To Craig Whetter, for always being there for me.

Jack Fitterer, for believing in me since high school. Thank you for your friendship.

To Betty Bonnet for her wonderful mentoring, coaching and encouragement throughout the years.

To my sister, Scooter, and my brother, David, for all your guidance all these years. To my cousins, Denise Vincent and Dennis Porter for their constant faith in me.

To three ladies who have inspired me with their own strength of mind and resiliency through their personal dilemmas, Shanna Axelson, Shan Luvisa, and Wendy Cariello.

To Bill and Jackie Stringham, the best in-laws a person could ask for. Your generosity of your time and energy is priceless. Thanks for being there for Darcy and I. We love you both very much.

Finally to my parents, Dave and Ida Madrid. Your parenting and advice has guided me to where I am today and where I will go tomorrow. I love you both.

In Memory of
Dan Stringham
1956-2006

CONTENTS

PREFACE

We live today in a global economy characterized by rapid change, accelerating scientific and technological breakthroughs, and an unprecedented level of competitiveness. These developments create demands for higher levels of education and training than were required of previous generations. Everyone acquainted with business culture knows this. What is not equally understood is that these developments also create new demands on our psychological resources. Specifically, these developments ask for a greater capacity for innovation, self-management, personal responsibility, and self-direction. This is not just asked at the top. It is asked at every level of a business enterprise, from senior management to first-line supervisors, and even to entry-level personnel.

A modern organization can no longer be run by a few people who think and many people who merely do what they are told. Today, organizations need not only a higher level of knowledge and skill among all those who participate, but also a higher level of independence, self-reliance, self-trust, and the capacity to exercise initiative—operating at a high level of personal responsibility.

It is easy in the high-stress environment of today to imagine that we are controlled by forces over which we have little or no control. It is easy to see ourselves as victims and to explain our disappointments or misfortunes in terms of the malevolence of "the system"—or the universe. For those who feel tempted to view their life that negatively, or some aspect of it—as parents or as CEOs, as spouses or as managers, or as salespersons, or as teachers, or as members of a team—*Get over It and Get on with It* is a wake-up call.

It tells us that so much more is possible than we had thought possible—but not if we permit our dreams to remain only dreams.

Jim Madrid and Joyce Quick, M.A., M.S.W.

The power of living self-responsibly is the basic theme of this book, and of Jim Madrid's inspiring and imaginative program, *The Ten Principles of Entelechy*. "The curriculum we teach," he writes, "has been shaped by many minds, starting with Aristotle, who coined the word *entelechy*. It draws heavily from the work of prominent researchers in cognitive, organizational, and behavioral psychology, as well as from a wealth of real-world experience."

Get over It and Get on with It does not assume that its readers see themselves as losers—on the contrary. It assumes that most have lives that work, personally and/or professionally, at least in some areas. It also assumes that most of us have dreams, aspirations—*goals*—which we have failed to achieve, and wonder why there is such a gap between performance and fulfillment.

"Our happiness depends on ourselves," wrote Aristotle, and Jim Madrid, taking this idea and running with it, is a pleasure to behold.

Nathaniel Branden

INTRODUCTION
WHAT'S IN THIS BOOK, HOW TO BENEFIT FROM IT

My Past and This Book's Purpose

You may not be particularly interested in knowing that I grew up in White Center, Washington, near Seattle. We called it Rat City; I'll spare you the details. You may not care that today, my family and I live in a wonderful place—Orange County, California—in a community my childhood buddies might have dubbed Fat City. Obviously, my circumstances have changed, and I don't just mean where I live. For several decades, *everything* in my life, personally and professionally, has been getting better. These days, I walk around with an incredible sense of well-being and gratitude—a smile lighting up my face and a glow doing the same for my heart.

Even if my past doesn't matter to you, I hope those last two sentences are of interest, because creating a better life is what *The Ten Principles of Entelechy* education is about. It's what my company and this book are about, too. Your job/career, relationships, health, finances, family, connections to community, feelings of contentment, energy level, and satisfaction—all can be improved greatly.

I don't mean to suggest that your life is currently a mess. If that is the case, this book can certainly help, but chances are you're doing fine. Maybe not as well as you could be, but all things considered, okay. Of course, I thought things were okay back in Rat City, too. At least I did for a while.

I had a mother who fiercely believed in the mercy of God, the value of family and the virtue of hard work. Mom was one of Nordstrom's first children's shoes salespeople, and she set an example I've always tried to live up to. My father was, and still is, as outgoing as they come. He taught me to treat strangers as friends I haven't yet met a concept he says Will Rogers stole from him! And I had siblings, aunts and uncles who, despite all our quirks and quibbles, gave me oceans of affection and praise.

As I grew older, I also had the constant turmoil, frustration and negativity that seemed to be part of that environment at the time. It wasn't a great place to grow up. I wanted to make a good life for myself, but wasn't sure how to do it. My future looked uncertain at best, not something I felt even slightly excited about. Then, in high school, I reached a turning point. I had a physical education teacher and coach who understood cognitive psychology.

They're Only Life-Changing Ideas If You Live Them

The coach told us that when it came to creating success and achieving goals, nothing, no accident of genes, good looks or family wealth, had more impact than our own thoughts. It had always been part of the wisdom of the ages, he said, but now there was scientific research to prove it.

Thoughts made people successful? How could that be? I always figured it was exactly the things he mentioned—money, looks, and luck—that determined why some people made it, while others lost out. What's more, he said that we could achieve just about any goal we wanted, if we knew how to control our thoughts. He taught us a few simple "mind control" techniques, such as watching our self-talk and using affirmations and visualization, and he made sure we practiced them. Next thing we knew, we were starting to win more games. Not only that, our grades began to improve, and we were doing better at home with our parents. I could hardly believe how good it felt, knowing this stuff. The future started to look like it was filled with interesting and exciting possibilities!

Eventually, our coach quit because he wanted to teach people how to use this information on a larger scale. The corporation he started became very successful, with branches in Europe and Australia. I worked with him for several years, facilitating training sessions and consulting with business leaders who wanted to use this information to benefit their employees. I worked with nonprofit organizations, too—at-risk kids, college athletes, and community groups—many wonderful people all over the globe.

One of the most important lessons I learned during those years was that understanding and talking about these concepts is relatively easy. The real challenge is living them—assimilating them so that they become second nature—and applying them in everyday life. I knew that if I were going to rise to that challenge and take charge of my own destiny, I had to be willing to take a big risk. I had to leave the sheltering umbrella of my ex-coach's organization and strike out on my own.

THE TEN PRINCIPLES OF ENTELECHY: CHANGE YOUR MIND, CHANGE YOUR LIFE

Fast forward a few years. Founded in 1997, Entelechy Training & Development is the name of my company and *The Ten Principles of Entelechy* is our flagship seminar. The curriculum I teach has been shaped by many minds, starting with Aristotle, who coined the word *entelechy*. It draws heavily from the work of prominent researchers in cognitive, organizational and behavioral psychology, as well as from a wealth of real-world experience.

Along the way, Entelechy's educational process has expanded and gained clarity through several inspiring collaborations and a great many highly perceptive clients and seminar participants. It has been profoundly influenced by the work of Dr. Nathaniel Branden, who has been called the father of the self-esteem movement, and one of the great psychologists of the twentieth century. He has been a good friend and mentor to me over the past few years.

I share and uphold Dr. Nathaniel Branden's definition, "Self-esteem is the disposition to experience oneself as competent to cope with the basic challenges of life and is worthy of happiness." Further, let us acknowledge that virtually all the material on self-esteem I present here is based on or derived from Dr. Branden writings.

The Ten Principles curriculum and related programs are now used by thousands of individuals and organizations, here and abroad. It is still something I try earnestly to live, every day. In fact, I firmly believe that living *The Ten Principles* is the reason why my situation is as good as it is, why it keeps getting better, and why I experience the joy of a life blessed by the spirit of abundance.

At the core of this education is one simple, profoundly important truth: Your thoughts and beliefs are played out and reflected in your life. *If you change your beliefs, your life changes accordingly.* In other words, when you improve what's going on inside your mind, what's happening outside it improves, too—automatically and often quite dramatically.

Once again, this is not really news. From Aristotle to Norman Vincent Peale, from Napoleon Hill to Dr. Phil, those who saw the immense power of these ideas have tried to get the rest of us to see it, too. But even if you can understand and accept these concepts, the "how" of applying them may not be obvious. After all, this isn't something most of us are taught in school, unless we're psychology majors. It isn't usually something we learn at a parent's knee, either, and, honestly now, how many of us read Aristotle?

A WORD OF THANKS AND AN ASSURANCE
Thank you for choosing this book, and for being curious enough to read this far. You may be wondering if it will be worth your time to continue reading. No matter who you are, or whether you have heard of *The Ten Principles of Entelechy*, I am certain the answer is an unqualified yes.

Thousands of people have used *The Ten Principles of Entelechy* to change their lives for the better. These people come from almost every conceivable field, industry, background and circumstance. As a result, I have unshakable confidence in the ability of this information to serve as a powerful catalyst for growth.

I believe you will find a number of things in these pages that will be immediately useful. You will discover ideas that generate insight, concepts that inspire creativity, and suggestions that lead to greater confidence and well-being. You will find other things that take time to assimilate and practice, but if you persevere, I have no doubt that you will be well rewarded.

I can't guarantee that you will do better or feel better after reading this book, because, as you might expect, there's more involved than just reading. But I can comfortably predict that if you use even a small portion of its contents on a daily basis, you'll be glad you did. Your personal and professional relationships will improve, as will your ability to set and achieve goals of every kind. You will be able to move steadily toward the life of abundance and fulfillment you most want. Now and then, you will even be able to take great leaps of progress. What's more—and this is of growing importance in our rapidly changing, ultra busy, highly competitive world—your stress level is likely to decrease.

CLOSING THE GAP BETWEEN POTENTIAL AND PERFORMANCE

I wrote this book to help people get over it, whatever "it" may be, and get on with living fully and successfully. "Get Over It and Get On With it" is far more than a catch phrase. Although it may sound simple, it is at the heart of what I teach and central to the concept of personal and professional growth. It offers a proven and effective way to, in effect, "update the human operating system."

Within these pages, you will find a collection of easy-to-learn, easy-to-live concepts that can enable anyone—no matter how educated or unschooled, how wealthy or poor, how sophisticated or simple—to change their thoughts and their lives.

In other words, *it reduces the gap between potential and performance.*

Throughout the book, you will find questions and exercises designed to expand your self-awareness or demonstrate the application of a concept. A reading list has been included at the end. It includes many of the works upon which *The Ten Principles* was based, as well as several that expand upon the concepts I present. The art and science of personal growth makes for fascinating reading; I hope that what you discover in these pages will inspire you to learn even more.

Part I is a condensed version of *The Ten Principles of Entelechy* education. Although it is abbreviated, it includes all the essential information that seminar participants receive. Each chapter presents one principle. I suggest you read them in order, as some concepts will be easier to understand in light of what has gone before.

7

If you are a *Ten Principles* graduate, don't skip Part I because you're already familiar with the material. Repetition is one of the ways your brain's neural pathways become stronger. Reviewing Part I will reinforce your ability to quickly recall and gain access to these powerful concepts. What's more, you may find that something you had previously missed will jump out at you, or a new application for the concept will become clear.

Each chapter in Part I begins with an Overview, which describes what you can expect to learn. Each concludes with several thought-provoking questions to help you identify exactly where you want to grow.

Part II explores how *The Ten Principles* can be applied to benefit you in your personal life. This section covers your relationships with significant others—spouse, family, children, friends, neighbors, and loved ones—as well as health and fitness, personal finances, and emotional stability.

Part III is all about improving your professional life. Whether you're self-employed, working for others, unemployed, in transition, or a student preparing to build a career—this section will help you use The Ten Principles to create positive change, including change at the organizational level.

Part IV focuses on your spiritual life. It concerns your connection to something I like to call The Greater Good, whether you view that as entirely human or inspired by something divine. It is also about the spirit of generosity that gives rise to a life of *abundance,* in the finest sense of the word.

What You can Expect

You will get much more from this book if you complete the exercises and answer the questions. Don't simply imagine that you are doing them. Get out a pen or turn on your computer and take a few minutes to record your thoughts.

If what you read leaves you hungry to learn more, log on to our web site, www.getoveritandgetonwithit.com, where you will find a wealth of additional information, products and services to help satisfy your appetite. If you are moved to share what you have learned, great! But remember that most of us dislike being force-fed, so take it easy. Temper your energy and enthusiasm with tact and good timing.

THE CHOICE IS YOURS

You can read self-help books, go to seminars, listen to audios and watch videos until the cows come home, but if you are unwilling to do the work of change, you won't see results. You will keep going from book to book, seminar to seminar, and you will keep searching for the "right" one—the one that will finally work magic for you.

But there is no fairy godmother, and no one is going to show up with a magic wand. No one can change the quality of your life but you. Getting the right job, the right house, the right spouse, the right car or the right body won't do it. Reading the right book won't do it, either— not if you don't change your habits, attitudes and beliefs.

A man goes into a bookstore and asks the clerk, "Where's your self-help section?" The clerk says, "Well, sir, if I told you that, it would defeat the purpose!" This silly joke brings a smile and makes a point. I can give you the benefit of decades of experience in the human potential field, and I can paint as vivid a picture for you as I can of the benefits you will realize if you choose to change. But you and you alone have to take accountability for actually changing your thoughts and your behavior, and for making those changes stick.

ACCOUNTABILITY JUMPSTARTS CHANGE

I urge you to accept that accountability. The moment you do, the change process is set into motion. When you take 100 percent responsibility for the quality of your life, and once and for all, stop being a victim, you put incredible power into your own hands. *Get Over It and Get On With It*. You will then welcome challenge, because challenge will make you stronger. You will take failure in stride, because you know it has important lessons to teach. You will discover that your only enemies are those who make you forget your purpose, harden your heart, or stop growing. And you will discover that your allies are everywhere.

By the way, I am convinced that accountable people are happier and have much more fun. When you're no longer a victim, and you know you can weather any storm, you can relax. You become confident and optimistic—a person for whom smiles and laughter happen naturally and frequently.

A Prayer for Each Reader

May the entelechy inside you lead to fulfillment and abundance. May you challenge yourself and rise to meet it, again and again. May failure teach you, and success bring you great rewards. May you find the process of learning and using *The Ten Principles* as exciting as the end results. And may the changes you set into motion—because of what you read here—put a glow in your heart and a smile on your face—every day of your life, starting now. God bless you.

PART I
THE TEN PRINCIPLES OF
ENTELECHY

These Ten Principles of Entelechy will give you the tools to deal with life's everyday challenges and assist you in living your life on purpose. You will have the process by which you will be able to enhance any part of our life: Health and fitness, relationships, career, personal finance, spirituality, business, fun, family you name it and this process will help you achieve the vision that you have for the future. But just like any diet, the one that works is the one you use and maintain.

Enjoy the journey!

Principle One: Take Change by the Hand

To live is to change; to live fully is to change often.

Overview: Change—The First Principle of Life
The first of *The Ten Principles of Entelechy* is the first principle of life itself. Whether it is the kind that *happens to you,* generated by outside forces, or the kind *you make happen,* change is the only thing that's constant over time.

Even if you find nothing in this principle that you don't already know, it will remind you of several important concepts that set the stage for what's to come. If some of what you read is new to you, great! It will serve an equally important purpose. Those "Ah-hah!" moments when your mind opens to an idea are the seeds of growth. They generate a new consciousness and creative energy.

When you've finished reading this chapter, you will:

- Realize that change is a constant experience, and one that presents both challenges and opportunities.

- Recognize the ways in which people respond emotionally to change—whether it's change forced upon them by external forces or generated internally.

- See that minimizing the "down time" often associated with change is a great advantage.

- Have a foundation for acquiring skills to help deal constructively with change in every aspect of your life.

WHAT'S NEW?

Every living thing changes constantly. You are not the same person you were ten years ago. You're not even the same person you were ten minutes ago! Everything that's not alive changes all the time, too, although it may be harder to see. In this principle, I will focus on how change affects people.

At work and at home, we are all forced to deal with change. Today our families face the negative effects of 9/11, global warming, Chinese capitalism, and premeditated mass murders on campus. Even good things have been changing very quickly—for us as individuals and families and for us globally. Thanks to a computer-driven technology explosion that began a few decades ago, and is picking up speed all the time, the rate of change is so fast it's downright amazing. It can also be unsettling.

WE ALL HAVE BECOME HYPNOTIZED BY OUR ENVIRONMENT!

We see it at work, in ultra high-speed systems that control communication, ordering, invoicing, accounting, inventory and record keeping; analyze results; predict profits; and develop new products. We have higher standards for customer service, new competitors and markets, and innovations in nearly every aspect of business. We see it at airports and many other public places, and we see it in the international community as it tries to develop strategies to defeat terrorism and come to grips with the new reality of globalization.

We see it at home, too. Electronic shopping and banking, computers in classrooms and on kitchen counters, and a vast number of options and choices we've never had before are revolutionizing our personal lives.

Watch yourself as you go through your day. Notice all the things you do differently now than you did five years ago, one year ago, last month, last week, or even yesterday. Incredible, isn't it? If you think things changed more slowly when you were a kid, you're right. And if you find yourself longing for those good old days, you may be in trouble.

CHANGE EQUALS STRESS, BUT HOW MUCH?

If you feel uncomfortable with the amount and rate of change, you're not alone. Change creates a certain amount of stress for everyone. You may like some of the changes you see and you may dislike others, but the process of transition is usually stressful, even if it's a change for the better. Often what you may find yourself wishing for is simply a time-out. Too much change equals too much stress.

For some people, change of any kind, and in any amount is incredibly stressful. They oppose it and complain, resist it and ruminate, defy it and develop stress-related symptoms. Examples of people who don't handle change well are all around you. No doubt you know several of these folks personally. From time to time, maybe you are one.

It's not surprising that so many of us feel threatened by this tidal wave of change. It's never happened before. We aren't equipped to deal with it. It makes us nervous, irritable, and even panicky. There's nothing in our experience that we can draw from for a script to follow. We're not sure whether it's going to help us or hurt us, and we can't quite understand how to control it.

No wonder so many people bury their heads in the sand and try to ignore it, or decide it's a destructive force and try to fight it. Or, they adjust when they absolutely have to, but spend a lot of time reminiscing about the "good old days."

For another sort of person, though, change, except for rare events such as terrorist attacks, isn't scary at all. On the contrary, it's stimulating and empowering. These people take change in stride and look for ways they can take advantage of it. They see change as an ally, not an adversary. They focus on how change will benefit them—not on the losses it will bring. Many even enjoy and look forward to change.

CHANGING YOUR MIND ABOUT CHANGE

If benefiting from and enjoying change doesn't sound much like your current reality, don't worry. That, too, can change. This first principle is based on the premise that how well you handle change depends on the way you think—on your attitudes, beliefs and expectations. Fortunately, you can learn to control the way you think. You can learn to think in ways that let you take change by the hand, before it takes you by the throat!

15

Principle One lays the groundwork for the other nine principles and for your own personal change initiatives. It begins the process of learning to think in ways that allow you to quickly adjust to change, deal constructively with obstacles and achieve the goals you want to achieve, no matter what you encounter along the way. In other words, it is the foundation for *Getting Over It and Getting On With It!*

FIVE STAGES OF ADAPTING TO EXTERNALLY-IMPOSED CHANGE

The book *On Death and Dying*, grew out of Dr. Elisabeth Kübler-Ross's famous interdisciplinary seminar on death, life, and transition. In this remarkable work, hailed as one of the most important psychological studies of the late twentieth century, Dr. Kübler-Ross explored the five stages people usually go through when facing the reality of their own imminent death or that of a loved one.

I have found these stages to be remarkably similar to those we experience when facing change that is imposed on us. Not that I want to compare the loss of a loved one to somebody stealing your stapler off your desk, but human nature is what it is.

The five stages are:

1. **Denial.** At first, we tend to disbelieve or deny that the change has taken place. This stage may last only a few moments or much longer. "This can't be happening! If I ignore it, maybe it'll go away."

2. **Anger.** We feel furious at the person/organization that imposed the change on us. We may be angry with ourselves, too, even though we couldn't have stopped it. "This change is stupid and I hate it! It'll never work! I'd like to give them a piece of my mind!"

3. **Bargaining.** We make deals with God or the powers that be. "If I do just this much, can I avoid most of the hassle and stress? Can I just pretend I support this and get by with not really changing?"

4. **Depression.** We feel miserable or numb, although anger may remain under the surface. If it continues long enough, the depression may require treatment. "What's the point of even trying? I'll never adjust and it'll just get worse."

5. **Acceptance.** Our resistance has tapered off. Now we simply accept the reality of the change. "Okay, I guess this change is for real. I'm going to make the best of it, whatever that takes."

Later in Part I, you'll learn proven and effective techniques that can help minimize the "down" time associated with the first four responses. They will allow you to advance quickly to acceptance, to *Get Over It*, the stage that allows you to move on, to learn from the experience and grow. That's exactly what I mean when I say, *"Get On With It."*

Five Stages of Self-Directed Change
Change that originates internally—in other words, change you choose and direct yourself—typically involves a different set of experiences, such as:

1. **Pre-contemplation.** We have no intention to change. We may be unaware or under aware that there is a problem or fail to see the benefits of change.

2. **Contemplation.** We know that a problem exists and are seriously thinking about overcoming it, but have not yet made a commitment to take action.

3. **Preparation.** We intend to take action soon, so we develop a strategy and/or enlist support to prepare for the change process.

4. **Action.** We do what it takes to modify our behavior or environment in order to solve the problem. We give the change our time and energy.

5. **Maintenance.** We work to prevent a relapse into an old behavior and consolidate the gains we attained during the action stage.

As you read more about *The Ten Principles,* you'll also learn how to manage these stages so that the changes you most want can be created quickly and smoothly.

ATTITUDE SHAPES MEANING

Whether change is imposed upon you by external forces or you initiate it yourself, one thing is always true: it's your *attitudes, beliefs* and *expectations* that determine the role change plays in your life and whether it works for or against you.

Some people think that their attitudes, beliefs, and expectations are an unchangeable part of who they are, like their eye color. Fortunately, that's not so. Beliefs, attitudes, and expectations are no more permanent than the way you wear your hair or what you eat for breakfast. You acquired your belief system gradually, as you grew up; it took years. That's fortunate, because what is learned can be unlearned. This time, the learning can be entirely self-directed and entirely beneficial.

YOUR BELIEFS SHOW UP IN YOUR LIFE

As you learn more about *The Ten Principles of Entelechy,* I hope you will be willing to take a good look at your beliefs, while keeping an open mind. If you do, you will discover some fascinating things about yourself. In fact, what you'll see when you examine your beliefs is a reflection of your life.

For example, if you believe that life is a struggle, you spend a lot of time struggling with one situation or person after another. If you believe that money is hard to come by, you have trouble making and/or keeping it. If you believe that you are a great salesperson, you close sales and cash commission checks while others are complaining or making excuses.

There is simply no way you can live a life that is different from your core beliefs. Whether it is your relationships, career, finances or even your physical health, your beliefs about the kind of person you are and the way these things work will show up. It's no mystery why this happens. *Life mirrors your beliefs because your beliefs determine your behavior.*

As you examine your beliefs, think about and answer the following questions:

- How well are you able to control your thoughts? How critical are you of yourself and others?

- Do you see any benefit in "retiring" some of your beliefs and adopting more useful ones?

- Do you want to keep doing things the way you've always done them because it's less stressful? Or, would you like to investigate some new approaches that may yield better results?

- Would you like to become a confident explorer in an ever-changing world? Or, do you turn to the past for the comfort of "been there, done that" and the illusion of certainty?

- Are you willing to view change as an adventure that can lead to the life you've always wanted?

- Are you on your way to getting over it and getting on with it?

By the time you have finished reading this book, you will know how to change your beliefs, if you choose to. You will have techniques at your disposal that will allow you to develop attitudes that help rather than hinder you. I think you will be surprised at how easy it is! All you need is your own amazing mind along with the principles and processes you will learn as we go along.

REFLECTIVE QUESTIONS

1. What's changed for me in my personal life during the past year? How have these changes affected me? How do I feel about them?

Change   How It Affects Me   How I Feel About It

2. What's changed for me at work during the past year? How have these changes affected me? How do I feel about them?

Change   How It Affects Me   How I Feel About It

3. In general, have I learned to see change as good or bad? Who were the role models that probably caused this attitude?

4. If I could change one thing about myself (not counting things that can't be changed), what would it be?

5. If I could change one thing about my job, what would it be?

樂

PRINCIPLE TWO: OPEN YOUR EYES AND YOUR MIND

WHAT YOU SEE IS MOSTLY WHAT YOU LOOK FOR.

OVERVIEW: HOW AN OPEN MIND IMPROVES YOUR EYESIGHT

Could you be holding onto some of your beliefs and behaviors because you just can't see a better way? In this chapter, you will learn that what you see or otherwise perceive is largely what's important to you. This is true because of something called the reticular activating system, or R.A.S. Your R.A.S. is a network of cells located near the base of your brain. It is constantly scanning your environment for two kinds of information: 1) things that are valuable, or, 2) things that represent a danger or threat. If something is important to you for one of those reasons, your R.A.S. will make sure it gets through to your awareness. If it's not important, you're likely to miss it. If you do notice it, you're likely to quickly forget.

As a result of reading this chapter, you will:

- Realize that we all have a highly effective network of brain cells called the R.A.S. that screens out unimportant information.

- Understand the basics of how the R.A.S. works, as well as how goal setting activates it.

- Recognize how stubbornly locking onto one idea limits perception and causes us to lock out a wealth of information.

- Know what *scotomas* are and see how we build them with our beliefs.

- Understand the relationship between scotomas and the R.A.S.

THE RETICULAR ACTIVATING SYSTEM: YOUR BRAIN'S SPAM FILTER

The function of your R.A.S. is something like the work done by a computer's spam filter. An incredible barrage of sensory data comes at you all the time, 24/7—sights, sounds, smells, movements, and sensations. If you had to pay attention to all of it, you'd be completely overwhelmed and unable to act. Your R.A.S. prevents this sensory paralysis from happening. It allows you to perceive and focus on the things that are most important. At the same time, it lets in everything you need to ensure your own safety and well-being. But this highly efficient system that usually promotes your best interests can also work against you.

For example, if you're absolutely convinced that something is true, you may ignore information that could prove it false. If you firmly believe there's only one right way of doing something, you probably won't even consider suggestions that lead to other methods. If your mind has locked onto one idea, you put up barriers to other possibilities.

LOCKING ON, LOCKING OUT

Has anyone ever called you stubborn? Do you occasionally think of yourself as stubborn? If so, are you secretly a bit proud of it? Of course, stubbornness has advantages and disadvantages. It's certainly good to refuse to abandon your principles, give up on yourself, or quit trying when something is really important to you. It's good to stubbornly persist in your efforts to achieve a goal that truly matters to you.

But the wrong kind of stubbornness can cause trouble. It will keep you locked into ways of thinking and behaving that are not in your best interest. It will close your mind to ideas that could bring you more success and happiness. And, perhaps most importantly, it will stop you from growing.

Why does being stubborn sometimes have such a negative, and limiting effect? Why is it so important to keep an open mind most of the time?

It comes down to this: *what you see is mostly what's important to you.* You have seen the truth of this yourself, again and again. After coming home from the mall one day, my wife, Darcy, said, "There sure are a lot more pregnant women out there than there used to be." No surge in pregnancies had caused her observation. Darcy, who was expecting our first child, had simply never noticed them before.

If you are in the market for a new TV, advertisements for TVs will jump out at you whenever you read the paper or go shopping. If you are thinking about buying a house, you'll spot "For Sale" signs by the dozens when you're out for a drive. If you are trying to lose weight, anything that has to do with weight loss will jump out at you—nutritional supplements in the supermarket, articles in magazines, TV commercials, and people talking about it across the room at parties. It isn't that these things weren't there before. They were in front of you all the time. But they weren't important, so your R.A.S. screened them out.

Scotomas: Self-Created Blind Spots

A computer operates according to the instructions given by its programming. Similarly, your R.A.S. screens out information according to your beliefs. For example, if you are convinced that something is true, your R.A.S. will tend to keep out information that might prove it false. You build a *scotoma*—a sensory blind spot—to it, and the scotoma causes you to literally block it out. It's the reason why Darcy missed those other pregnant women, or why you missed the "For Sale" signs.

Here is an interesting example of a certain type of scotoma. Read the sentence below and count the number of F's you see. Read it once again and verify your count. Don't skip to the next paragraph until you have finished.

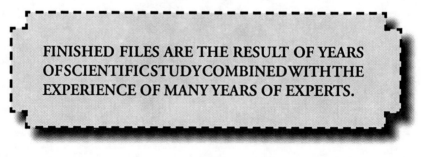

FINISHED FILES ARE THE RESULT OF YEARS OF SCIENTIFIC STUDY COMBINED WITH THE EXPERIENCE OF MANY YEARS OF EXPERTS.

How many F's did you see? Most people count three or four, but there are actually seven. You probably missed the word "of." This exercise always makes a few jaws drop when we do it in our *Ten Principles* seminars. No one can believe they got it wrong. How could they possibly miss something so obvious, and so simple? But most of us miss those F's at first. We don't hear the F in "of" because it has a V sound. This is especially true if we were trained to read phonetically. In our minds, we hear a "V" so we promptly build a scotoma to the fact that it's actually an F. We quite literally don't see it.

Don't feel foolish if you counted wrong at first. Your mistake has nothing to do with your IQ and everything to do with your conditioning. The first time Jim saw this exercise, it was in a book of puzzles for kids, and he had to look up the answer at the back!

Old Cowboy, Young Cowboy

Here's another example. In the picture below, is the cowboy young or old? Would it surprise you to know that the drawing contains *both* images? At first, most people can only see one of them, no matter how hard they try. After they are shown how to find both images, the scotoma is forever gone.

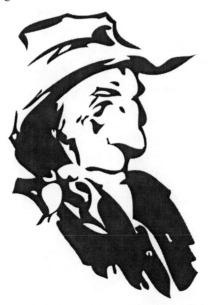

If you still can't see both, ask someone who can see both to help you.

The Key to Busting Scotomas and Opening Your Mind

If you believe that you are not good at something, you will have no trouble finding ways to avoid it or fail at it. If you believe there is no satisfactory solution to a problem, it will be easy for you to find reasons to support your belief. In fact, "good" reasons will be everywhere you look. What you probably won't notice, though, is any evidence to the contrary. Whenever you believe that there is only one truth, one way, or one answer, your mind won't waste energy on trying to discover something else that might work. You will find lots of "good" reasons to ignore or devalue suggestions from other people, too.

The proverb, "Argue for your limitations, and sure enough, they're yours!" has it right. That is what overly stubborn people do. As a result of early learning or conditioning, they have decided what's true for them, and they have locked onto their beliefs. Accordingly, their R.A.S. makes it almost impossible for anything that doesn't support their bias to get through.

Fortunately, all it takes to open a closed mind is the decision to do it, and a bit of practice. If you are genuinely willing to see new truths, then new truths will get through. If you are sincerely interested in finding better ways to live, then better ways will soon become evident. When you deliberately keep your mind open and your goals clear, you will put your powerful R.A.S. to work for you.

Are You Ready?

Another old saying predicts that, "When the student is ready, the teacher will appear." That's one way of explaining what happens when you decide to put aside your limiting beliefs and open your mind. When you are ready and willing to learn, the entire world becomes your teacher.

Does this mean that if you deliberately open your mind, you will be overwhelmed with a tidal wave of information? Will you go into some sort of sensory overload and start burning out brain cells? Of course not. You will still notice and remember things that are threatening or valuable. However, an open mind allows your R.A.S. to expand what it lets in. It gives you instant access to a wealth of new information.

When you open your mind, you open all your senses. When you break free of your conditioning, you see things you never saw before. You hear about things you didn't know existed, make connections you never imagined, meet people who can help you, and do things you never dreamed you could do. You grow by leaps and bounds because you have access to vast quantities of information that you had locked out in the past. Your world becomes bigger, richer, and more fulfilling

USE IT OR LOSE IT

Your brain is capable of handling everything that you declare to be important. It's similar to a muscle—the more you use it and push its limits, the stronger and more capable it becomes. The less you use it, the more it weakens and the more difficult it is to do even routine tasks.

Opening your mind to new information in this way, doesn't mean you have to change any of your core values. If you want your R.A.S. to function as effectively as possible, be clear about what those values are. Remember, whenever you declare something to be important, your R.A.S. starts scanning for anything that is of value or a threat. Thus, the clearer you are about your values, goals, and vision for the future, the easier it will be for your R.A.S. to alert you to helpful information. Your R.A.S. is, in essence, a program that helps you to update your human operating system. It functions much like the message you get on your computer: Updates are ready to be installed.

The Balance Wheel exercise at the beginning of Part II is designed to help you clarify your values. Later in Part I, I will talk about techniques that can help you do the same thing. When you stop being vague about what's important to you, and start being crystal clear, you'll automatically be putting the amazing power of your R.A.S. to work!

REFLECTIVE QUESTIONS

1. Do other people ever call me stubborn, or do I think of myself as stubborn? In what areas? What might happen if I let go of some of my stubbornness?

2. Do I know any people who have scotomas to things I can see clearly? Who are they? What are they blind to?

_____Person   **What Can't They See?**_____

3. Have I ever had a scotoma that caused me to miss something important? If so, what?

_____**When?**   **What Couldn't I See?**_____

Principle Three: Understand How Your Mind Works

We are just beginning to understand and learn how to use the incredible power of our brains.

Overview: How You Create Your Self-Image

Isn't it a shame that your brain doesn't come with operating instructions? Most of us have at least a basic grasp of how our bodies function, but we know very little about how our minds work—even though it's just as important to our health and well-being. The more you understand about why and how you perceive and process information, make decisions and behave as you do, the better able you'll be at making choices that lead to success and happiness.

This book cannot possibly tell you all there is to know about how your brain works—that would take a library filled with books. But it can focus on a couple of key mental processes and help you learn how to take charge of them. Why would you want to do that? If the changes you want to make in yourself and your life are going to last, you must change your beliefs about yourself—your self-image. When you change your beliefs, you *automatically* change your behavior—and when behavior changes, so do results.

Once you've read this chapter, you will"

- Have a better understanding of the way your brain works by looking at the conscious, subconscious, and creative subconscious processes.

- See why it's difficult, if not impossible, to behave in ways that conflict with your self-image.

- Realize that we all make decisions based not on our potential, but on our past experiences.

- Understand why changing your beliefs is necessary in order to achieve lasting changes in your behavior.

YOUR AMAZING BRAIN

During the last few decades, more new information about the brain has come to light than during the last few centuries! We are only now developing the technology that allows us to effectively study the brain—an amazingly complex organ. Your brain regulates and controls everything that goes on in your body. What's more, it stores memories, creates dreams and fantasies, regulates language, and generates the chemical reactions you experience as emotion.

The brain is often compared to a computer—a kind of living bio-computer, with a virtually unlimited capacity. Like a computer's processor, results depend on hard wiring and programming. If you remove an old program or insert a new one, the same computer that controls the missiles on a nuclear submarine can design business cards or play solitaire. Tweak input slightly, and results change. Sometimes they improve, and sometimes they deteriorate.

You know a few things about how your body functions, but like most of us, you have probably been taught little or nothing about how your brain operates. You may have picked up some basic psychological principles from the popular media, but that doesn't always give an accurate picture. When it comes to understanding how your mind works, you may not have much more than old wives' tales and personal experience to go on. Let's try to change that right now. Here, in a nutshell, are a few facts you should be able to put to good use as you learn to direct your own growth.

THE SYSTEM CALLED "MIND"

Your mind has three aspects or functions that dramatically affect the quality of your life. They are interdependent and have no clear boundaries, but we usually discuss them separately for ease of understanding.

Conscious. The part of your mind that deals with your awareness. Among its functions are:

1) perception, through the senses—*What's this?*; 2) association with the past—*Have I seen anything like this before?*; 3) evaluation—*What happens now? How does this affect me? Should I do something?*

Subconscious: The part of your mind that operates outside your awareness. This is a vast storehouse of memories, feelings, images, and reflections. Everything you've ever experienced or felt is recorded here. The subconscious is thought to be immense compared to the much more limited conscious mind.

Creative subconscious: This is the part of your mind that makes sure you act like the person you subconsciously believe yourself to be. It plays a role in problem-solving and generates drive and energy to resolve differences between your beliefs and current reality.

These three aspects of mind will figure prominently in the material I'll cover later.

KEY CONCEPTS FROM YOUR BRAIN'S OPERATING SYSTEM MANUAL

Knowing something about how the conscious, subconscious and creative subconscious work gives you a great advantage in managing your own growth and development. The more you know about how you make decisions and why you behave as you do, the more you'll be able to make choices that lead to more success and happiness. That is why Principle Three spotlights two critical ideas:

1. **You automatically associate and evaluate new situations based on the past.** You unconsciously ask yourself, "When have I seen something like this before?" "When have I been in a similar situation? What do I already know about this that I can use now?" This extremely rapid, generally unconscious process helps you to function efficiently. It allows you to retrieve information and apply or adapt it to new situations. That way, you don't have to "reinvent the wheel" every day of your life.

Sounds good. So what's the problem? Just like being stubborn, this process has both up and down sides. It may often remind you of negative associations from your past. Consequently, it can keep you from having an open mind about the present and future. For example, if you're invited to a party where you won't know anyone, you'll probably decide whether to go by evaluating similar past experiences. Were they terrifying, exhilarating, or neutral? Did you meet pleasant people and make valuable contacts? Or, did you go home feeling it was a waste of time or worse? You'll also factor in your beliefs about yourself, based on the past. Do you see yourself as congenial, unattractive, boring, outgoing, shy, or curious? How well do you believe you function in social situations like this?

2. **You act like the person you believe yourself to be.** Self-image is the sum-total of your beliefs about yourself, based on your interpretation of past experience; it governs much of your unconscious behavior—another highly efficient system. You don't have to think about how to behave like yourself, do you? You automatically do it. Because it is based on the past, your self-image may be keeping you "stuck in a rut." You may be behaving in ways that no longer serve you, bring you happiness, or represent the person you most want to be. If so, it may be time to change some of the things you've been telling yourself about who you are.

THE TRUTH OR *YOUR* TRUTH?

Most of us think we have a handle on the truth, and most of us think we're doing the best we can in terms of goal achievement. During the past few decades, however, behavioral scientists have conducted enough research to set us straight.

- **We act in accordance with the truth *as we perceive it to be.***

- **We set our goals *based on our beliefs,* and not on our potential to achieve.**

For thirty-seven years, I bit my fingernails to the quick. I was embarrassed by my ragged nails and inflamed cuticles. I tried countless times to stop, but the "quit" never lasted. Nothing worked—not the bitter potion mom painted on my nails, and not my dad's hand-slaps and impatient admonitions. My self-image was solidly that of a nail-biter, even as an adult. Before I could stop biting my nails, I had to adjust my self-image.

I used visualization and affirmation techniques to strengthen my new belief. My favorite affirmation was, "I have attractive, well-manicured hands." (Chapter 8 explains how affirmations work to change beliefs.)

Soon, my behavior began changing to match the words. While driving home one sunny spring afternoon, I decided to stretch my comfort zone by going into an upscale nail salon—even though I was nervous about revealing my hands. The manicurist was friendly and sympathetic. The process didn't take long, and my nails looked great! Soon, I began to have manicures regularly. Before long, my affirmation became more deeply imprinted, and I stopped biting my nails completely. The habit just fell away. My hands became a source of pride.

REDUCING YOUR BAGGAGE TO CARRY-ON SIZE

No matter what your hands look like, and no matter what your present circumstances or situation, *The Ten Principles* can help you control some critical mental processes. They give you tools you can use to override obsolete negative programming so you can stop making choices based on fear, anxiety and self-doubt.

Imagine how your life would change if you started to make decisions based not on the negative experiences you've had, but on the positive experiences you want! Imagine what might happen if you behaved like the person you *want* to be, rather than the person you *used* to be! *The Ten Principles* enable you to use your amazingly powerful mind to bring you success rather than frustration, happiness rather than conflict, and confidence rather than doubt.

Change your beliefs and you change your behavior. Change your behavior and you change results. It won't feel strange or stressful. It won't feel like you're trying to be someone else. It will feel completely normal and natural, like you've put down a lot of heavy, unwieldy baggage. You'll feel lighter and more centered because you'll be changing from the inside out—the best way to be sure that change is comfortable, and the only way to be certain that change lasts.

REFLECTIVE QUESTIONS

1. What are some things I've been reluctant to try at work because of negative past experiences?

2. What are some things I've been reluctant to try in my personal life because of negative past experiences?

3. What kind of person am I? Here are a few adjectives that describe the way I see myself:

Positive traits   Negative traits

_____   _____

_____   _____

_____   _____

_____   _____

_____   _____

4. How difficult is it for me to behave in ways that oppose these beliefs?

5. If I believed I could not fail, what might I do:

   at work:

   in my personal life:

Principle Four: Adjust Your Explanatory Style

The way you explain the world determines how you experience the world.

Overview: Optimistic Self-Talk is a Skill You Can Develop
Explanatory style is simply the way you interpret and attempt to understand yourself and the world around you. Another term for explanatory style is self-talk.

If your self-talk is largely pessimistic or negative, you can literally talk yourself out of success. If it is generally positive or optimistic, you have a definite advantage. Optimists tend to get results that reflect their attitude. They achieve more than pessimists do at work, school and on the playing field. They bounce back from setbacks more quickly and feel depressed less often. They have happier, more satisfying relationships, better general health, and may even live longer. Makes you wish you could be more optimistic, doesn't it? Well here's some good news. You can.

The concepts in *The Ten Principles of Entelechy* and the information in these pages teach the skills of on-purpose optimism. When you gain control over your self-talk, you can upgrade your self-image. This is an incredibly valuable skill, because *we move toward and become like what we talk and think about.*

When you've finished reading this chapter, you will:

- Understand what explanatory style is and how it shapes your self-image and behavior.

- Realize how explanatory style influences your personal and professional success and well-being.

- Understand the benefits of becoming an optimist and the disadvantages of being a pessimist.

- See how controlling your self-talk helps you develop a positive, optimistic explanatory style and a stronger self-image.

SELF-TALK DETERMINES EXPLANATORY STYLE

Explanatory style is something you learned and developed over time, starting when you were young. It is positive or negative, optimistic or pessimistic, depending on your self-talk. The term "self-talk" may sound as if you're having an actual conversation with yourself, but that's not usually the case. While some self-talk is aloud, most of it is silent, and in the form of thoughts. It happens rapidly and automatically. You're not usually aware of it, and it goes on almost all the time.

Self-talk is directly connected to your beliefs. While you were growing up, you formed a belief system about how the world works. You also developed a constellation of beliefs about the kind of person you are. These we call your self-image. Over time, you developed an explanatory style to match and mirror your beliefs.

Optimists tend to see the silver lining in dark clouds, focus on solutions instead of problems, and look for the best in themselves and others. When things go wrong, they don't waste time blaming themselves and feeling miserable. Instead, they minimize the down time, increase their efforts, and confidently expect improvement. Sure enough, they usually get improvement. Not surprisingly, a great many high-performance people are optimists.

FIFTY THOUSAND THOUGHTS A DAY

All day long, our brains are busy chattering away, creating endless self-talk. It has been estimated that the average adult thinks about 50,000 thoughts a day! Most of those thoughts are about—you guessed it—yourself! This means that except when you are occupied with something that demands concentration, you spend most of your time thinking about yourself.

While self-absorption is not something you necessarily want to encourage, self-awareness is. Every time you have one of those 50,000 thoughts, you have an opportunity to do yourself a favor by framing it in a positive way. First, it requires your awareness. Every day, thousands of things go right for you. You take most of them completely for granted. You don't give them a first, let alone second thought. What about the two or three things that go wrong? They get a huge amount of your attention, don't they? Sometimes you can't seem to stop thinking about them, even though almost everything else in your life is operating with amazing smoothness and stability.

FIFTY THOUSAND OPPORTUNITIES FOR OPTIMISM

Even though most of your life is good, how many of your thoughts are critical instead of grateful? How many times a day do you judge yourself, put yourself down, compare yourself unfavorably to others, blame yourself, belittle yourself, or tell yourself you're not measuring up? How many times every day do you call yourself lazy, slow, dumb, fat, ugly, boring, confused, clumsy, second rate, or any of a host of other belittling things? Do you tell yourself that those negative judgments are the truth? Can you easily and quickly point to evidence that supports your explanation?

Instead of a handle on the truth, what you have is a death grip on some negative conditioning. Think about it. Those low opinions you have of yourself didn't start out in your own mind. Most were given to you by other people—parents, teachers, older brothers and sisters—anyone who was an authority figure to you when you were growing up. Were these devaluing opinions true even then? It's doubtful. They were simply reflections of someone else's negative conditioning.

WHERE DID ALL THAT NEGATIVITY COME FROM?

If you currently believe that you are lazy or selfish, or hold onto any other negative label, think back to the first time you remembered hearing that opinion. Who did it come from? How often did you hear it? How did you *learn* to see yourself, not as you had the potential to be, but from a negative, critical point of view?

Habitual negativity is learned behavior. If you were fortunate enough to have parents who loved, respected, encouraged and praised you a lot, you probably still feel good about yourself most of the time. That positive self-concept is the foundation upon which *self-esteem* (your opinion of your worth) and *self-efficacy* (your opinion of your competence) are built. When you were growing up, every bit of praise, loving gesture or word of encouragement was like a brick in that foundation, making it steadier and more solid.

THE BAD NEWS

On the other hand, every critical comment or belittling gesture was like a wrecking ball. Whenever you were devalued, treated as if you didn't matter, or absorbed someone's message that you were deficient, it took a little chip out of your self-image. Bit by bit, you learned to see yourself in a highly critical way, and you saw the world in the same way. You became a pessimist, without ever intending it.

Even if you didn't get a lot of critical, negative attention when you were growing up, chances are you had some limiting labels hung on you. Those labels affected your explanatory style. Later, after you became an adult, you didn't need anyone to remind you to act like the deficient person you believed yourself to be; your subconscious took on that job. You gradually internalized the negative messages and labels you heard so often as a kid. Today, your self-talk echoes them.

This isn't a problem when it comes to positive images. On the contrary. When you've internalized mainly positive messages about yourself, your self-talk reflects these messages. You have the optimist's advantage. On the other hand, the negative messages you've internalized caused nothing but trouble. A negative, pessimistic explanatory style leads to negative perceptions, negative behavior, and negative results. It's a kind of self-fulfilling prophecy. These negative messages limit you in ways you may be unaware of. They keep you locked into a behavior that causes disharmony, lackluster performance, and further erosion of your self-esteem.

THE GOOD NEWS

Fortunately, there's good news, too—very good news. With the help of the information from this book and *The Ten Principles of Entelechy*, you will soon learn how to turn off your negative tapes. You'll be much more aware of negative, and critical self-talk, and you will be able to stop it from doing more harm. You will be able to control your self-talk and adopt a more constructive, optimistic explanatory style.

A REVEALING EXPERIMENT

Make a note of the time. Starting right now, censor yourself. Do your best to be aware of every negative, critical, pessimistic, fearful, belittling or devaluing thought that goes through your mind, and whenever you notice one, nip it in the bud. Don't let anything negative linger in your mind or come out of your mouth. Stop any and all forms of negativity. This means no sarcasm of yourself, no putting yourself down, no joking or belittling of yourself or of anyone else for the next twenty-four hours.

You'll probably be surprised at just how much negative self-talk you'll catch during that time. I hope you will also begin to see what a great benefit it can be if you clear most of it out.

OPTIMISTS ARE NOT PERFECTIONISTS

You may never become perfect at stopping all your negative thoughts, but perfection isn't the goal. It's true that optimists expect to do well, and they generally do. But they don't expect perfection from themselves or anyone else. In every endeavor, at any given time, there can be only one Number One. At the Olympics, there is only one gold medal winner in each event. When, despite their best efforts, optimists lose, they don't come unglued. They acknowledge their disappointment and get back to work, trusting they'll have another chance down the road. They can relax and enjoy being one of the many who know they tried their best, whether or not they won the gold.

In other words, optimists are not driven to succeed, no matter what the cost. If careful analysis of the situation calls for it, they're okay with letting go and moving on. Giving up has a bad reputation in some people's minds, but the truth is that winners sometimes intentionally quit and quitters sometimes end up winning. As the old country song says, the challenge is to "know when to hold 'em and know when to fold 'em." Because they tend to be more relaxed, hopeful, and confident, optimists can make either a "hold or fold" decision work for them, depending on which makes sense at the time.

OPTIMISTS: WIN OR LOSE, MORE PRODUCTIVE, RELAXED, AND HAPPY

Almost without exception, people who make these techniques an integral part of their lives report results that just keep improving. In the same way, *The Ten Principles* have enabled organizations of many types and sizes around the world to operate more productively, profitably, and harmoniously.

Soon, you will be able to put these powerful principles to work in your own life. In just minutes a day, you can silence the critical, pessimistic inner voice that stops you from doing all you can do, and gives center stage to your internal optimist. Your attitude toward life will change and new behavior will naturally follow. Next thing you know, you will be getting the kind of results optimists get—the kind of results you may once have thought were impossible.

REFLECTIVE QUESTIONS

1. What kind of explanatory style did my parents have? Were they optimists or pessimists?

2. What's the explanatory style where I work? What's my explanatory style while I'm at work?

3. How self-critical am I? When do I give myself a hard time about mistakes or not measuring up?

4. When I fail to meet my own standards, how do I usually explain it to myself? When I exceed my own standards, how do I explain that?

Principle Five: Expand Your Comfort Zone

Growth always requires you to do things you've never done before.

Overview: Expanding Your Comfort Zone Improves Self-Image

For all of us, some situations or experiences are perfectly comfortable, while others are not. We feel at ease working or talking with certain people, but avoid interacting with others. We are relaxed and confident when participating in some activities, but dislike it when we have to get involved in others. Being relaxed and comfortable is pleasant, so we tend to enjoy the people and experiences that make us feel that way. Even if we don't actively take pleasure in them, we're at least neutral, and not at all "on edge" or anxious.

What happens, though, when we must venture outside our pleasant, and familiar comfort zone? How does it feel when we are expected to socialize with people who seem very different from our usual circle of friends? Or, what happens to us if we are thrust into a completely new work or social setting, or we attempt to learn a complex new computer program, or make a bunch of cold calls? What about being asked to do something we associate with painful past experiences?

For most people, the answer is tension and stress. Whenever you are required to operate outside your comfort zone, all you want to do is get back to it so you can relax. No wonder it can sometimes be such a struggle to motivate yourself or anyone else to change. It doesn't even necessarily matter what the benefits of change are likely to be, either. If it means trading ease and comfort for tension and stress, it's usually a tough sell!

For many of us, it is such a white-knuckle experience to operate outside our comfort zone that we habitually avoid anything new and different. It's so much easier to stick with the old and familiar! The more successful we are at avoiding the stress of new experiences, the less successful we will be at growth. It doesn't matter whether it's personal or professional, intellectual or emotional, growth always means risking, stretching and venturing into new territory. The key is to learn how to do those things while minimizing the associated stress.

By the time you have finished reading this chapter, you will:

- Know what comfort zones are and how they affect your feelings and performance.

- Realize that your self-image always regulates the size of your comfort zones.

- Recognize why you feel tense or anxious when you try to behave differently, go places you've never gone to before, or attempt new activities.

AT EASE IN THE ZONE

Remember, your self-image is the way you see yourself, consciously, and more important, subconsciously. It's a collection of beliefs you've developed over time concerning who you are, what you're like, what you deserve, and how you behave. Some of these beliefs are about when and where you feel comfortable, and when and where you feel out of place.

Has this ever happened to you? You walk into a restaurant, shop or even someone's home, and you immediately feel or say to yourself, "This is my kind of place!" What you're saying, in other words, is, "I fit in here." That's because the setting matches or complements your mental picture of who you are and what you're like. It's inside your comfort zone.

No doubt you've experienced the same thing when getting to know new people, attending or participating in various events, and in many other situations. When you feel that way, you're *in the zone*. As long as you stay inside it, you feel relaxed, at ease, and relatively free from anxiety. Even if they're technically new to you, things seem familiar. You're confident that you can handle whatever comes up. You can relax and be yourself. You have no worries about trying to change your normal behavior.

WALKING THE PLANK

Imagine a ten-foot-long, six-inch-wide plank placed flat on the floor. If I offered you twenty dollars to walk across it, you probably wouldn't hesitate. It would be easy. You'd feel quite comfortable. But what if that same plank were raised high in the air and stretched between two skyscrapers? What if I raised the pay to $1,000.00, or even $100,000.00? It's likely that no amount of money would motivate you to walk across at that height. Possibly no reward I could come up with would tempt you to try it. Even the knowledge that you're perfectly *capable* of doing it wouldn't matter. It's simply too far outside your comfort zone. What changed? The only thing that changed was the four inches between your ears. You see fear instead of reward.

The further outside your comfort zone you go, the more uncomfortable you get. Can you remember how you felt the first time you went out on a date? What about your wedding ceremony or your first day on a new job? What was it like the first time you ever made a presentation or speech before a large group? Or, took a trip to the hospital for surgery? Or, even attended a party where you didn't know a soul?

These were not "business as usual" experiences for you at the time, and if you're like most people, you were definitely not relaxed going into them. You may have noticed sweaty palms, a pounding heart, tightness in your chest, muscle stiffness, and rapid or shallow breathing. If you weren't conscious of feeling a lot of tension while the experience was actually happening, perhaps you noticed it afterward. Did you breathe a long, deep sigh of relief? Crave a nap? Want to pop a cork to celebrate? One thing is almost certain. You were very happy when you could get back to your normal life—happy to be who you are without having to think about it. It's human nature to feel like that. We much prefer operating within our comfort zones to walking the plank.

Have you ever brought personal items from home to decorate an office or cubicle? Made excuses early to leave a party where you felt out of your depth? Have to stop yourself from tidying up someone else's desk? Quit a job because you didn't feel at ease around the people? Whenever you find yourself forced outside your comfort zone, you'll do everything you can to: 1) get back where you belong, or 2) change the situation so it's more like what you feel comfortable with.

COMFORT ZONE AND SELF-IMAGE

If your self-image is outgoing and social, you will feel comfortable around other people and in social settings. If you see yourself as a leader, you will be calm and relaxed when it's time to take charge. If you believe you have to struggle for success, you may feel anxious when things go too smoothly. If you think you are a quick learner with plenty of ability, you will feel at ease when you need to master a new skill. If you see yourself as slow and clumsy, you'll probably falter, fumble, and make mistakes.

This almost goes without saying, but should be said anyway: Comfort zone and self-image are directly connected. The higher and stronger your self-image is, the broader your comfort zone. Neither is cast in stone; both are possible to change.

IMPROVED SELF-IMAGE EQUALS BIGGER COMFORT ZONE

You have grown. So has your comfort zone. You currently feel perfectly relaxed and comfortable with many things that once caused discomfort or stress. Have you ever resisted buying something because you couldn't see yourself owning it, and now you can't imagine living without it? Have you ever avoided a fashion or style because it wasn't you, but down the road it felt just right? How comfortable did you feel when you first tried to operate power tools or drive a standard shift car? What about now? How about public speaking? If you've done it a lot, did it get easier over time? Did it once make you nervous to even think about taking on the role of parent, spouse, or supervisor—and now that you've done it, it doesn't seem so daunting? Your comfort zone has changed due to those experiences. So has your self-image.

In light of this, two things are clear: 1) The stronger and higher your self-image, the broader your comfort zone, and 2) The broader your comfort zone, the easier it is for you to grow.

GROWTH EQUALS EXPANDING YOUR COMFORT ZONE

Growth always requires stretching your capabilities. It means trying new things and venturing into new territory, often without a map. Growth means expanding the limits of your comfort zone, too, because when you're growing you're doing more and being more than you ever have—until you get used to it. Then it feels perfectly comfortable—perfectly normal—second nature. You've assimilated the new behavior and expanded your comfort zone.

Do you see how valuable it is to have a broad comfort zone? Expanding your comfort zone improves your ability to grow and achieve your goals. Can you imagine what might happen if, instead of anxiety, tension, and stress, you felt anticipation and excitement when you moved outside your comfort zone? If your comfort zone was so broad, you could go anywhere, meet anyone, do anything you chose to do, and still feel relaxed and comfortable.

That's what *The Ten Principles* and this book are designed to facilitate. They offer solid science and tested techniques to expand your comfort zones in every area you choose, with a minimum of tension and stress. Using this information and these techniques, you can grow in ways you may never have imagined possible.

With an expanded comfort zone, new experiences can feel exciting, and not threatening. Instead of stressful, they can be satisfying. Instead of making you want to hurry back to the couch, they can inspire you to seek out bigger, and bolder challenges. You will be able to face those challenges with confidence, knowing that even if accomplishing them is a bit beyond your ability right now, with persistence and patience, you can grow into them.

REFLECTIVE QUESTIONS

1. Where or when do I feel out of my comfort zone at work?

2. Where or when do I feel out of my comfort zone in my personal life?

3. When I was growing up, what did I learn from my parents about venturing outside my comfort zone?

4. Can I remember a time when stretching my comfort zone really paid off for me? What happened?

PRINCIPLE SIX: EXERCISE YOUR IMAGINATION

IMAGINATION IS ONE OF YOUR GREATEST GIFTS AND STRONGEST ALLIES.

OVERVIEW: YOUR IMAGINATION CAN HELP YOU SHAPE A NEW REALITY

When my son, Chase, was still a little boy, we were having a conversation about the difference between things we imagined and things that were real. Chase said he thought that imaginary things were what came after the words, "What if."

Although the dictionary's definition is slightly different, Chase was essentially right. Imagination is the mind's blueprint for constructing reality. Every man-made creation who has ever been brought into the world first existed as a thought—a "what if" inside someone's imagination. We traveled in wheeled carts or on the backs of animals until someone dared to imagine the internal combustion engine. We were earthbound until someone dreamed up a vehicle for flight. We communicated over distance by handwritten missives until the telegraph, telephone, fax, and Internet were invented. However, before they could be invented, someone had to imagine them. First came the idea, or vision; then came the reality.

Your own life is no different. What you can do is limited largely by your ability to clearly imagine it. That's why your imagination may be the most wonderful gift you possess. If you can mentally picture yourself behaving in a certain way, it is far more likely that you will actually behave that way. The more clear and vivid your mental picture, the easier it is to bring it to life.

You don't have to worry about *how* that transformation will happen. The Wright brothers weren't sure how to build an airplane, but they believed they could figure it out. Edison wasn't certain about the kind of filament that would allow him to create a controlled light source from electricity, but he knew that if he persisted in searching, he would find it.

It's the same process that will work for you, and it doesn't matter what your goals are. Be clear about what you want, imagine it repeatedly, and believe in your ability to invent the reality as you go along. That belief is called *self-efficacy*. When your self-efficacy is strong, you know that if it's possible, you'll do it. Your self-efficacy and your imagination are like muscles. The more you exercise them, the stronger they will become, and the more good things you'll be able to create.

When you've completed Principle Six, you will:

- Recognize the immense power of the imagination as a creative force.

- Be aware of five things high-performance people do that make it much easier for them to achieve their goals.

- Learn why end-result thinking is a critical part of the goal achievement process.

YOUR GREATEST GIFT

Aside from a few physical constraints, what you can do in life is limited mainly by your ability to imagine and believe in it. If you can clearly and vividly see yourself behaving in a particular way, achieving something you want, or feeling a certain emotion, it's far more likely that you'll do it. *Belief begets behavior, and behavior creates results.*

This is nothing new or unusual. In fact, you are already using your imagination all the time, whether you're conscious of it or not. "I think I'll fix myself a tuna salad sandwich on toast" is the idea that arises in your imagination to stimulate the actual sandwich creation. "I want a better job, and one where I feel appreciated" is the idea that comes to you before you start the job search. "I need to work late tonight to get this report finished" precedes the reality of staying at your desk past quitting time.

FIVE GOAL-ACHIEVEMENT HABITS OF HIGH ACHIEVERS

Form follows thought. Your ideas are like melodies playing in the mind of a musician before he or she sits down at the piano and makes them into music other people can hear, too. Your ideas have the potential to be transformed into reality, depending on whether you decide to act on them and what form that action takes.

I have found that high-performance people (high achievers in their chosen fields) tend to use their imagination in five specific ways to create goal achievement. Their goals are:

1. Clear and specific

2. Written and reviewed often

3. Described as end-results in present tense

4. Realistic—neither too easy nor too difficult

5. Described and mentally experienced as if they were already real

You will learn more about these five habits of thought and behavior, as well as how to incorporate them into your life, as we move ahead.

WHAT YOU *THINK ABOUT* IS WHAT YOU *BRING ABOUT*

Most people have little or no understanding of how to control their imaginations. They have never really given it much thought. When they have a knotty problem to solve, they usually concentrate on the problem, but the harder they try, the more stuck in the problem they get. The pictures they create in their imagination are of what's wrong instead of what it would look and feel like if it were right. How can they create a solution if they can't imagine a solution? Why do they seem so surprised to see problems all around them when problems are all they see inside their minds?

There is nothing magic or mystical about this. Your most frequent thoughts and deepest beliefs about reality affect your perception and behavior. Your perception *is* reality to you. My perception *is* reality to me. What is the truth? It's hard to say. Scientists agree that it is impossible to separate human perception from so-called reality. Your truth depends on your environment and experiences. What is true for you here and now may not be true at all for someone else in another time, another place, or another culture.

CAN YOU CHANGE YOUR BELIEFS?

Can you deliberately change your perception of the truth? Can you change what you truly believe? Of course you can. You have already changed your mind about numerous things in your lifetime. No doubt, you can think of dozens without difficulty. In the past few decades, many people have altered their beliefs about diet, exercise, job security, divorce, child rearing, alternative medicine, money management, the stock market, defense spending, and global warming, to name just a few. Along with new information and experience come new beliefs.

Similarly, as we begin to imagine new possibilities, they become more likely. Gradually, in most cases, and suddenly in a few, they become our new reality. If you are still doubtful, remember Christopher Columbus. He was able to imagine a world beyond the horizon, where the vision of most everyone else stopped. As he acted on his imagination, and his beliefs about what was possible, he changed the world forever. Many visionary individuals are doing the same today.

THE MORE YOU USE IT, THE BETTER IT WORKS

If you want to grow and develop both personally and professionally, your imagination can be a tremendous ally or an overwhelming obstacle, depending on how you use it. Fortunately, the more accustomed you become to using it, the more you can do with it. This concept goes far beyond positive thinking. It involves deliberate, and positive mental *experiencing!*

Remember the last time you had a nightmare? Did your body understand that the experience was "just a dream," or did your heart pound, and your breathing speed up? Did you feel actual fear before you woke up? How long did it take that feeling to go away?

Now call to mind a sad event from your past. Close your eyes for a moment and take yourself back to that time. Recall what it felt like, looked like, sounded like, and even smelled like. If you imagine it vividly enough, you may find yourself feeling sad again, perhaps even moved to tears, even though nothing remotely like it is actually happening.

An everyday example involves what happens when you're really hungry and you imagine something you'd love to eat. Does your stomach start to rumble and your mouth begin to water?

These are examples of your powerful imagination at work, creating an emotional or physical experience that isn't actually happening, but nevertheless feels completely real. Amazing, isn't it?

IMAGINATION MULTIPLIED BY VIVID EQUALS REAL

As far as your subconscious mind is concerned, anything that you vividly imagine is just as "real" as if it had actually happened in the world outside your mind, especially if it stirs your emotions.

A formula that makes it easy to remember this concept is:

$$I \times V = R$$
(Imagination times Vividness = Reality)

You will learn more about this important concept when we talk about Principle Eight. You will also explore ways of putting it to practical use, personally and professionally, later in the book.

INVENTING THE HOW

The Ten Principles of Entelechy teaches scientifically sound methods for expanding the horizons of what you can see yourself doing and being. As you progress through this book, I hope you will begin to want to set bigger goals for yourself. Like Columbus, you won't have to know exactly *how* you will achieve them, either. That's one of the best things about this process.

If you clearly imagine what you want and your self-efficacy causes you to believe you are capable of achieving it, you will figure out how to do it. Even though you may have many questions and few answers right now, you will find them. Remember your R.A.S.? As soon as you decide that a goal is important, you start to see all sorts of things you never noticed before. Your mind opens up to new information, new ideas, new sources of help, and new ways to do what you want to do. You become very energized and resourceful. Once you are firmly committed to the goal, *you will invent the how* as you go, using your creative and powerful imagination!

REFLECTIVE QUESTIONS

1. When I was a child, was I encouraged to exercise my imagination? If so, how?

2. Are there times when I allow myself to daydream, without feeling that I should be doing something more active and obviously productive? If yes, how often do these times occur and how long do they last? If no, why not?

3. Einstein once said, "Imagination is more important than knowledge." What do you think he meant?

4. When is your creative imagination most freely expressed? How does it affect your job when you are feeling imaginative and creative? How does it affect your relationships?

PRINCIPLE SEVEN: CREATE AND RESOLVE DISSONANCE

GROWTH THRIVES ON ENERGY GENERATED BY WANTING SOMETHING NEW AND FEELING DISSATISFIED WITH THE OLD.

OVERVIEW: MAKING COGNITIVE DISSONANCE WORK FOR YOU

Cognitive dissonance is a psychological term that may sound complex but is really quite simple. *Cognitive* refers to the thought process and *dissonance* is a kind of discord or conflict. Although we usually think of conflict as something to avoid, cognitive dissonance is a type of conflict that can be healthy and productive, especially when setting and achieving goals.

Whenever you vividly and specifically imagine something new for yourself—a better way of relating to your family, more rewarding career, greater financial security, improved physical fitness, record-breaking job performance, or anything else—you create cognitive dissonance.

That's because when you vividly imagine that new reality, you are trying to hold two "truths" in your mind at the same time.

1. The first is a picture of the reality you would like to create.

2. The other is a picture of your current reality—the way things are right now.

The conflict created by these two pictures causes cognitive dissonance. Like any other conflict, cognitive dissonance creates considerable stress. Your mind isn't wired to accommodate two different versions of the truth, and your body doesn't like all the stress that conflict generates. As a result, a tremendous amount of energy is generated to help you eliminate the stress and resolve the dissonance.

In this chapter, you will learn what it takes to relieve this stress. You will also see what a tremendously useful tool it is to be able to deliberately create and harness cognitive dissonance.

When you have completed this chapter, you will:

- Understand what cognitive dissonance is, what it feels like, and why it occurs.

- Discover the two ways in which cognitive dissonance can be resolved.

- Learn how to use the drive and energy created by cognitive dissonance to achieve goals.

THE HAMMER OF CONFLICT

You can't set a goal unless you first know what you want to accomplish, so imagining the new result, feeling, or condition, is the first step in goal setting. Whenever you vividly imagine something new for yourself, whether you know it or not, you also create a conflict. It doesn't matter what new condition you're imagining. It could be almost anything—a better job, better relationship, better appearance, better attitude, better bank balance—you name it. If you want something new and you imagine it clearly, you create cognitive dissonance

Dissonance is the opposite of harmony, comfort and smooth sailing. It makes waves, causes discomfort, and generates tension. These are feelings we usually prefer to avoid. There are times when conflict is not only unavoidable, it's also extremely useful. Conflict can be compared to a hammer—used in one situation, it can destroy or dismantle; used in a different way, it can help build or create.

COGNITIVE DISSONANCE IS NORMAL

It's important to realize that cognitive dissonance is a natural response to the kind of vivid imagining of goals we recommend. As soon as you start visualizing the change you want—as soon as you begin to clearly picture yourself doing things differently, living differently, and feeling differently—you can expect tension and stress to show up.

That is exactly what's supposed to happen. It is cognitive dissonance doing its job, as it should, whenever there is inconsistency between your beliefs and your actions or whenever your mental image of what's right for you doesn't match reality. It may not sound like much fun, but many high-performance people have learned to welcome it, stress and all, because of the tremendous creative energy it generates.

YOUR COGNITIVE CONSCIENCE?

Perhaps you can learn to welcome it, too, once you understand that cognitive dissonance is a good thing. In some ways, it is similar to your conscience. When you do something that conflicts with your moral or ethical standards, your conscience starts to do its job. It generates tension and stress, and perhaps even guilt and shame. These are very uncomfortable feelings. Sometimes they are downright painful, but they serve a purpose. They get your attention.

After they have your attention, what happens? Once you recognize that you're feeling badly, you may choose to override your conscience and ignore or lower your standards. You adjust your self-image downward to match your behavior. You are no better for the experience and even a bit worse, but the immediate stress seems to lessen. Doing this is like deciding to get rid of the scale because it tells you that your weight has gone up too far! In the long run, it doesn't serve you.

Ideally, your conscience will move you to do the right thing—make amends, resolve the conflict, and eliminate your discomfort by behaving like the person you know yourself to be. No doubt you would agree that you are better off because you have a conscience, even though it may make you uncomfortable at times.

CREATING DISSONANCE

You can also use cognitive dissonance to help you become a better person. Suppose your current reality is that you are thirty pounds overweight, but you really want to lose those extra pounds and regain your ideal weight. You look in the mirror and see your fleshy, rotund self. Then you close your eyes and vividly imagine the slim, fit self you once were and want to be again.

Before you even open your eyes again, the stress of cognitive dissonance will have started. Maybe you will be aware of it in your body—butterflies in your stomach, a feeling of tightness and dread in your chest, sweaty palms, or a bit of a headache building. Maybe you won't be conscious of it at all, but it will happen. Your mind cannot comfortably accommodate two conflicting versions of any truth or belief at the same time, especially your beliefs about who you are. You cannot see yourself as a slim, fit person, and still eat compulsively without generating stress.

Obviously, this concept has much wider application, going far beyond body image. You can't see yourself as a timid person and behave in a persuasive, outgoing way—not without creating discomfort and tension. You can't truly believe yourself to be kind and loving while behaving harshly or critically—not without dissonance. You can't see yourself as healthy and strong while neglecting your body's well-being—not without stress. These feelings are designed to get your attention and put you into action to resolve the conflict and eliminate the discomfort.

RESOLVING DISSONANCE

Resolving this uncomfortable conflict can be done in two ways. You must either:

1. Weaken/relinquish your picture of the ideal, and let it go in favor of your current reality.

2. Strengthen the ideal and bring it to life, causing it to become the new current reality.

Which are you more likely to do? That depends.

If your picture of current reality is stronger than your image of the change you want to create, then current reality will prevail. You will likely weaken or abandon your efforts to change, heave a sign of relief, or beat yourself up a little for giving up, and then return to the status quo.

On the other hand, if your vision of the change you want is stronger than current reality, change will win out. You will use the drive, energy and discomfort of cognitive dissonance to motivate yourself. You will become fiercely committed to making the new picture become dominant. You will be determined to do what it takes to create a new reality and evict the old one from your mind and from your life.

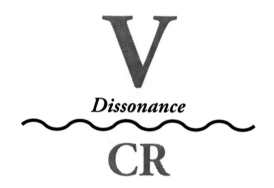

Dissonance

WHAT ARE YOU LOOKING FORWARD TO?

Perhaps one of the most valuable skills you'll learn from this book and from *The Ten Principles of Entelechy* is a scientifically sound technique that combines affirmative self-talk and imagery. This technique will allow you to harness the tension and stress of cognitive dissonance. In other words, you will be able to control it, instead of being controlled by it. You will know how to systematically strengthen your picture of what you want so that you can more quickly and easily bring it into reality.

In Principle Three, I described what happened to me when I began to experience cognitive dissonance around my habit of biting my fingernails. As I affirmed my image of myself with attractive, well-manicured hands, current reality began to change. The more I strengthened my picture of the new reality, the more my old picture of ragged nails and bleeding cuticles became obsolete.

If you practice this technique of affirming and visualizing change, you can become an expert at converting the stress and tension of dissonance into the drive and energy of goal achievement. When you combine this with what you have learned about how your mind works, comfort zones, explanatory style, the R.A.S., and the wealth of information you will find in the rest of these pages, there is virtually no limit to how much you can grow.

REFLECTIVE QUESTIONS

1. What am I dissatisfied with right now in my personal life?

2. What am I dissatisfied with right now in my professional life?

3. When I feel dissatisfied, how does it affect my stress level?

4. How much growing do I normally do during those times when my life feels pretty much the way I want it to be?

5. What does it feel like after I achieve a hard-won goal or complete a big project, but have no new goal in sight?

PRINCIPLE EIGHT: SAY YES TO YOUR FUTURE

THE POWER OF LANGUAGE TO FOCUS THOUGHT AND GENERATE EMOTION CANNOT BE OVERESTIMATED.

OVERVIEW: SPEED GOAL ACHIEVEMENT WITH AFFIRMATIONS

Principle Four focused on the benefits of controlling your self-talk and developing an optimistic explanatory style. Principle Six explained how to harness the immense power of your imagination. Combined, these two concepts can be used in a simple, systematic way to make goal achievement feel completely natural, even when the goal represents a big challenge. In this chapter, you'll learn a simple, yet powerful *affirmation* and *visualization* technique that can speed your goal achievement and help maintain motivation.

To affirm means to speak the truth—to make it more "firm" and real. An affirmation, then, is simply a statement that expresses a truth, conviction, or belief. Positive affirmations are tools you can use to become more like the person you want to be and achieve the goals you want to achieve. Some people prefer to call affirmations goal statements. Some prefer the term *mental imagery*. No matter what you call them, their purpose is the same—they make change easier by helping you improve your self-image.

How do affirmations work to upgrade self-image? Your subconscious can't tell the difference between something you vividly imagine and something that is actually happening. Used correctly and consistently, affirmations enable you to create mental experiences that are as powerful as the real thing, but even better, because they're completely under your control. It is like having the ability to practice a skill whenever you wish, but being able to practice *perfectly!* Imagine what that could do for your level of goal achievement.

In this chapter, I'll explain why affirmation combined with visualization works. I'll discuss how to create the most effective affirmations possible. I'll also talk about how to use them to solve real-life problems and create exciting, positive changes in every aspect of your life.

When you've completed this chapter, you will:

- Appreciate the importance of having goal statements or affirmations in written form.

- Know how visualizing your affirmations helps you change from the inside out—easily and without undue tension and stress.

- Understand why it is important to write goal statements as end-results that have already been achieved.

- Realize what it takes to become an "unconscious competent" at any skill, behavior, or attitude.

YOU ARE A CREATIVE GENIUS!

Human beings are creative creatures. You might even say, that by our very nature, we're all creative geniuses, because we all have the ability to transform thoughts into things that are real and meaningful. While we all have this innate ability, most of us do it unwittingly. Few people understand what it takes to do it *deliberately.* That's because most of us have never been taught the skills involved. We are largely unaware of our ability. We are filled with misconceptions about the creative process, and are easily deterred by obstacles and pitfalls. The results are predictably erratic and often disappointing.

Deliberate creativity may be a new idea to you, too, but it isn't hard to learn. Whether you are trying to create a work of art, a thriving business, a harmonious relationship, spiritual well-being, physical fitness, material wealth, or a more deeply satisfying life, the process is much the same. It happens through a progression of thoughts, words and deeds.

Transforming Ideas Into Reality

It's important to realize that thoughts, words, and deeds are not separate entities, as they may at first seem. Rather, they are completely interconnected. In the process of creating reality, each is a more "solid," and tangible form of the one that comes before. It may be helpful to imagine the progression like this: When steam cools and condenses, it becomes water. When water cools and condenses, it becomes ice—solid as a rock.

Your thoughts are like steam. They have a tendency to dissipate and disappear. Like steam, however, when contained and channeled properly, they are incredibly powerful. Just as steam can be used to drive mighty turbine engines, your thoughts are the drivers of almost everything in your life. They are the source of all your words and deeds, and the source of all your accomplishments, joys, and sorrows.

Words are the vehicles for moving your thoughts outside of your mind and into the world. They allow insubstantial ideas to take the first critical step toward transformation into reality. Just as water has more substance than steam, words have more substance than thoughts. Just as water can both create and destroy, your words have tremendous creative and destructive power.

When you use language in a systematic way, in the form of positive *affirmations*, and when you combine affirmative language with *visualization*, you make it much easier to create the reality you desire.

Affirmations: What They Are, and What They Do

Once again, to affirm means to speak the truth—to make it more firm, substantial and real. *An affirmation is a sentence or statement that expresses your belief about something, and it's your truth.* Affirmations contain words chosen carefully by you to help transform your goals into reality.

Affirmations can facilitate your efforts to create positive change and solve real-life problems, no matter how large or small those problems may be. Affirmations create and strengthen the thoughts, beliefs and feelings that lead to change-producing behavior. The words in an affirmation are very important. You must try to custom-design your affirmation so that it describes the end-result you want and adjusts your self-image in ways that help you create it. Remember, when your self-image changes, your behavior changes, too—automatically and without undue stress.

AFFIRMATIONS: PERFECT PRACTICE

Before I explain how to write and use affirmations, it's important that you clearly understand why they're so important. Since your subconscious can't differentiate between a "real" experience and one that you have vividly imagined, the words in an affirmation have just one function—to trigger vivid mental images and generate as much emotion as possible. When the picture is vivid and the emotion is truly felt, the visualized experience is recorded by your subconscious as the real thing.

Unlike the real thing, however, an affirmation is completely under your control. It's a type of mental rehearsal or practice, with one important difference—nothing depends on circumstance or chance. If you use them correctly, you can practice *perfectly,* every time, as often as you wish. Soon, having similar experiences in real life will no longer feel strange or stressful. Instead, it will feel perfectly natural, like something you have done many times before. Because, as far as your subconscious is concerned, you have!

In other words, systematic use of affirmations and visualization can help you become an "unconscious competent" at whatever skills you choose. You won't have to think much about it—whatever "it" is. Can you imagine what that kind of free-flowing, relaxed competency might do for your level of job performance? What about your financial stability, personal relationships, or even your health and fitness?

HOW TO WRITE A POWERFUL AFFIRMATION

Here are the eight essential steps to writing effective affirmations:

1. Affirmations are written in the **first-person, present tense**. They usually begin with the word "I," and they portray you doing and feeling something as if it were happening *right now.*

2. The words should **describe what you want**, but not what you don't want. Say, "It is easy for me to stay calm in stressful situations," not "I don't get upset when under stress."

3. Your affirmations should **describe actual achievement**, and not the possibility of it. Say, "I feel," and "I am," rather than "I can," or "I will."

4. Make sure your affirmations contain **emotion-packed words**. They should describe the good feelings attached to behaving in a certain way.

5. Make them **brief**—not more than one sentence long.

6. **Don't compare yourself to anyone else**. Don't affirm better performance than so-and-so. You are the only person you're competing with.

7. Similarly, **don't try to affirm change in anyone else** or control their behavior or responses.

8. Keep your affirmations **realistic**. Avoid words like "never" and "always." Strive for significant improvement, but not perfection.

NO SMOKE, NO MIRRORS

As you write your affirmations, remember that they are not magic. They are scientifically sound tools you can use to build a more positive self-image. They are not supposed to describe your present behavior or your present reality, even though you write them in the present tense. They are intended to describe a new reality *as if* it were true right now.

Does the fact that they aren't yet true make them misstatements or lies? Not at all. Affirmations accurately describe your potential—the behavior you want and the truth as you intend it to be. As I explained in Chapter Seven, this creates cognitive dissonance, which generates the drive and energy you need to bring your vision into current reality.

How to Use Affirmations: Read, Picture, and Feel

The process is neither complex nor difficult. All it takes is a few minutes a day and your full attention.

1. **Read.** Find a quiet place where you won't be disturbed for a few minutes. Take out your written affirmation and read it. If you have several affirmations, give each one ample time and attention. If one of them is a priority, give it a bit more time.

2. **Picture.** As you repeat the words, visualize the experience you are describing. Close your eyes, if that helps. Try to see yourself doing what you are affirming, in as much detail as possible. See yourself looking exactly as you will look, notice exactly what you will see. Put yourself in the center of the picture, as if it were a vivid dream. Use as many of your other senses as you can, too—hear it, move it, smell it, and feel it.

3. **Feel.** How will you feel once the desired result has been achieved and your mental picture has become real? *The effectiveness of an affirmation depends on the strength of the emotion it creates.* If you feel little or nothing when you say the words, the words will lack power. Be sure to put feelings into your mental picture. Will achieving your goal make you feel happy? Proud? Confident? Relaxed? Calm? Try to actually experience those feelings while you speak the words.

Remember the BAR Code

Bar codes are used everywhere these days to price and track every conceivable kind of product and process. You can use the letters BAR to remind yourself what it takes to bring your affirmations into reality.

B = Believe. Believe wholeheartedly in your ability to achieve the goal.

A = Affirm. Affirm the goal in emotion-packed words and vivid mental images.

R = Repeat. Stick with the process until you see results.

Affirmation FAQs

How long should my affirmations be?
Keep them brief—not longer than one sentence. Be as simple and specific as possible.

Can I work on more than one affirmation at a time?
Absolutely. I am usually working on half a dozen or more at any given time. However, don't create so many that you find yourself rushing through them or losing intensity and focus.

How often should I repeat and visualize them?
As often as possible without getting bored; aim for quality more than quantity. Once a day with good concentration is better than three perfunctory repetitions a day. Take at least thirty seconds for each. If you find yourself "getting lost in the feeling" of one particular affirmation, great! Go with it. You'll be cutting the time it will take to build drive and energy.

Is one time of day better than another?
Usually, I work on my affirmations for a few minutes every morning and evening. It may be different for you. Try to choose a time that will: 1) be open to you, day after day, and 2) provide the environment you need to focus fully.

How long will it take before I get results?
Affirmations work to help change your self-image. Small changes can happen very quickly; making deep changes to firmly entrenched habits may take longer. Remember, your subconscious doesn't know the difference between something you vividly imagine and something real. That's why your visualized experiences have nearly the same effect on your subconscious mind as your real-life experiences. You will get new results when you adopt new behavior. Affirmations make new behavior happen sooner and feel more natural.

How long should I keep repeating an affirmation?

When the change you wanted has been made and no longer requires much conscious effort, kiss that affirmation goodbye and write a new one. You may want to keep the old one around for a while, though. I keep a box full of "retired" affirmations that I look through now and then. It reminds me of how far I have come. Sometimes I take one "out of retirement" for a while, to be reinforced and refreshed.

How do affirmations work, again?

A handy formula to help you remember how affirmations work is I x V = R. Imagination times Vividness equals Reality. Because this is true, visualizing affirmations is an effective way to change your internal, subconscious picture—your self-image—your deepest beliefs about yourself. When you change beliefs, you change behavior, automatically.

Isn't it lying to affirm something as true if it hasn't happened yet?

When you repeat and visualize an affirmation, you are telling the truth about your potential. You're describing something you want to bring into reality as accurately and honestly as you possibly can. You describe it and visualize it as if it were true right now to make it real to your subconscious and create cognitive dissonance. In Chapter Seven, I talked about how dissonance generates drive and energy. Your affirmations are true, even if they haven't happened yet, and they are designed to be as effective as possible in helping you achieve your goals.

REFLECTIVE QUESTIONS

1. A problem I've been postponing solving (or a change I've been avoiding) is:

What unproductive/unwanted behaviors does this problem cause in me? What feelings does it generate?

Behaviors   **Feelings**

2. What would it look like if the problem were fixed, i.e., successfully solved? How would I behave? How would I feel?

Behaviors   **Feelings**

3. In *first-person, present tense,* write one sentence describing the end-result or outcome you want concerning this problem. Remember to use words that describe how you feel, too.

Sample Affirmations
Here are some of my affirmations.
(Borrow, customize, adjust and adapt to fit your goals.)

I am proud of the way I use affirmations and visualizations to make change easier and more comfortable.

I truly enjoy the few minutes I spend every morning and night repeating and visualizing my goals.

I love anticipating positive change as I work with my affirmations.

Repeating and visualizing my affirmations makes me feel strong, happy and confident.

It is exciting to feel my comfort zone expand as I affirm my own growth.

I love the increased energy and confidence I feel after affirming and visualizing my goals.

My self-image improves every day, along with my ability to enjoy life.

I aim not for perfection, but for steady improvement.

My self-talk is positive and my attitude is optimistic.

The more I use affirmations and visualization, the more I feel that I am truly in charge of my life.

Principle Nine: Strengthen Your Self-Esteem

The root of self-esteem is not achievement but those internally generated practices that, among other things, make it possible to achieve.

Dr. Nathaniel Branden, The Six Pillars of Self-Esteem

Overview: Six Practices That Build and Reinforce Self-Esteem
Few things are as important to our growth, development and happiness as high self-esteem. Even so, most people don't understand what self-esteem is, how it develops, or why it is so important.

First, let's lay a widely-held misconception to rest. People with high self-esteem aren't arrogant, self-absorbed, or in other ways "full of themselves." To put a complex concept simply, high self-esteem people are those who strive for more consciousness, have confidence in their ability to create a fulfilling life, and believe they have a right to succeed and be happy.

I share and uphold Dr. Nathaniel Branden's definition, "Self-esteem is the disposition to experience oneself as competent to cope with the basic challenges of life and as worthy of happiness." Virtually all the material on self-esteem I present here is based on or derived from Dr. Branden's writings. In his modern classic, *The Six Pillars of Self-Esteem,* people with low self-esteem tend to feel that they don't quite "measure up." As a result, they are easily manipulated by fear. They fear the collapse of their pretenses about themselves and the humiliation of failure, as well as the responsibilities of success. They are apprehensive about reality itself, in the face of which they feel inadequate. They face the basic problems of life with a pessimistic, self-defeating attitude, which contributes to an increasingly negative, shaky self-image.

How do people with high self-esteem get that way? While it is clear that certain qualities are genetically based, self-esteem is acquired over time and can be developed even after you are an adult. Your self-esteem is shaped both internally and externally, by your beliefs and behaviors, as well as the messages about yourself that you receive from significant others, organizations and your culture.

In this chapter, you will learn more about how strong self-esteem is developed. You will also read about six practices, that if you bring them into your life on a daily basis, will work wonders for your self-esteem and for the overall quality of your life. When you have completed this chapter, you will:

- Know what self-esteem is and is not

- Understand the six main ways in which self-esteem develops

- Begin to realize how building strong self-esteem can benefit you.

WHAT SELF-ESTEEM IS AND HOW TO BUILD IT
High self-esteem is not simply a matter of having a high opinion of yourself. If that were true, the most arrogant people would also be the ones with the highest self-esteem. It is not something you can develop simply by repeating affirmations, either, although affirming your strengths and abilities can be helpful.

Self-esteem is built by what you think and how you behave. The way you behave improves naturally as your self-esteem gets stronger, and your self-esteem improves when you behave in ways that strengthen it. Dr. Branden has written extensively about six ways to think and behave that strengthen self-esteem in *The Six Pillars of Self-Esteem* and elsewhere. I summarize his ideas for you here, but refer you to his books for more detailed information. (Please see Recommended Reading for a complete list.)

The Six Pillars of Self-Esteem are also *practices*. In other words, they are not simply ideas or concepts, but also actions carried out over time. They include:

1. **The Practice of Living Consciously.** To live consciously means that, whatever you are doing, and wherever you are, part of your mind is watching to ensure that your behavior is appropriate and aligned with your deepest values. It means that you accept responsibility for staying in touch with current reality and that you are aware of the possible consequences of your behavior. It means that you seek the truth and are open to new information, even when it may conflict with something you already think or believe.

Conscious living also means that you are aware, not only of what is going on around you, but also of what is going on inside you—your own thoughts and feelings.

If I brought 5 percent more consciousness to my professional life…

If I brought 5 percent more consciousness to my personal life…

2. **The Practice of Self-Acceptance.** Self-esteem and self-acceptance go hand-in-hand. You can't have one without the other. Self-acceptance means that you are willing to acknowledge and experience the truth of your own identity, without denial. You may not like some aspects of yourself right now, but you accept that they are there. You allow yourself to think what you think, and feel what you feel, both positive and negative. After all, you can't solve a problem that you don't admit exists.

In addition to being compassionate toward others, you are compassionate toward yourself, especially when you've behaved in ways that you regret or feel ashamed of. You do what you need to do in order to correct the behavior, but you don't beat yourself up about it.

If I brought 5 percent more self-acceptance to my professional life...

If I brought 5 percent more self-acceptance to my personal life...

3. **The Practice of Self-Responsibility.** You believe that you are the one who controls your life. You take responsibility for every aspect of your existence—your behavior and level of consciousness, goal achievement, use of time, the way you communicate, the quality of your relationships, and your own personal happiness and success. While it is true that you can't control everything that happens to you, you know that you can control your responses. You make a genuine effort to do so in ways that reflect your deepest values.

If I brought 5 percent more self-responsibility to my professional life...

If I brought 5 percent more self-responsibility to my personal life...

4. **The Practice of Self-Assertiveness.** You are willing to stand up for yourself and treat yourself with respect—to be who you are openly, and without apology. You are conscious of your wants and needs, and you honor them and express them appropriately. Self-assertiveness doesn't mean being aggressive, pushy or belligerent. It does mean speaking up when you have something to say and knowing that you are not here to live up to anyone's expectations but your own.

If I brought 5 percent more self-assertiveness to my professional life...

If I brought 5 percent more self-assertiveness to my personal life...

5. **The Practice of Living Purposefully.** You don't lose yourself in daydreams, wishes or hopes. Instead, you are clear about what you intend for yourself, and you work to make it happen. This practice is closely tied to your feelings of self-efficacy—your belief in your own ability to cause or make things happen, learn what you need to learn, and master realistic tasks or problems by persistence and effort. You set goals that have meaning for you. You follow through with actions to achieve them, and pay attention to outcomes so that you stay on track. You cultivate self-discipline, so you can postpone immediate gratification in order to attain a meaningful goal down the road.

If I brought 5 percent more clear sense of purpose to my professional life…

If I brought 5 percent more clear sense of purpose to my personal life…

6. **The Practice of Personal Integrity.** You live in ways that reflect your deepest values. You don't betray your own standards in order to be liked or gain approval from others. You don't spend a lot of time feeling guilty when you let yourself down or behave in a way that you regret. Instead, you acknowledge your actions and their consequences, make amends if possible, apologize if appropriate, and do your level best not to repeat the behavior. If the time comes when living by your standards seems to be leading toward self-harm, self-destruction or doing serious harm to others, you are willing to question those standards and revise them.

If I brought 5 percent more integrity to my professional life...

If I brought 5 percent more integrity to my personal life...

The Challenge and the Payoff

If you accept the challenge of integrating these practices into your life on a daily basis, you will strengthen your own self-esteem and create a framework within which you can feel good about yourself, *with good reason.* You will have confidence in the effectiveness of your mind, your ability to learn and grow, make good choices or decisions, and manage change. On the job and in your personal life, strong self-esteem is not simply something nice to have. *It is essential* if you're going to succeed and find fulfillment over time. Here's why:

- It helps you adapt quickly, without feeling threatened or doubtful, to constantly-changing conditions.

- It fosters a deep sense of responsibility and accountability, which will place you in good stead wherever you go, and in whatever you do.

- After a setback, crisis, or shake-up, it enables you to land on your feet and get back to work on what's important.

- It is the foundation for building mutually beneficial relationships—with family and friends, employers and employees, team members, and colleagues and coworkers.

Note: Nathaniel Branden, often called, "the leading pioneer in the field" of self-esteem psychology, is a Ph.D. psychologist, practicing psychotherapist, and best-selling author. His book, *The Six Pillars of Self-Esteem,* contains a wealth of information about self-esteem; I highly recommend it. I have asked his permission to use some of that information; he has kindly granted it.

REFLECTIVE QUESTIONS

When am I most likely to operate with a low level of consciousness? When am I most likely to operate with a higher level?

Are there specific things I do that weaken my self-esteem? What are they?

Are there specific things I do that strengthen my self-esteem? What are they?

What would be likely to happen in my professional life if I improved my self-esteem?

What would be likely to happen in my personal life if I strengthened my self-esteem?

PRINCIPLE TEN: ACCEPT ACCOUNTABILITY AND GET HAPPY

WHEN YOU PUT A SMILE ON YOUR FACE AND A GLOW IN YOUR HEART, YOUR LIFE WILL BE TRANSFORMED.

OVERVIEW: WHAT HAPPINESS IS, WHY IT LASTS, AND THE ACCOUNTABILITY FACTOR

What puts a smile on your face and a glow in your heart? Although some things consistently bring joy to a great many of us—children, family, sweethearts, getting lost in a pleasant activity—the answer is different for people of different ages, in different cultures, and circumstances. It's even different for you, depending on your surroundings, your health and energy level, what you're doing, and, most of all, what you're *thinking*.

Fortunately, you can learn to control what you think, at least to some degree. You can start today, right here and right now, by practicing *The Ten Principles of Entelechy*. If you really want more happiness in your life, you first need to accept the idea that no one can make you happy but you. Accepting personal accountability for your own happiness is critical to achieving it. With the possible exception of genetic influences, we are all 100 percent accountable for how happy we are, because we are 100 percent accountable for our lives—the parts we're proud of, and the parts we hide, along with the parts we like, and the parts we'd like to change.

With accountability comes power. Accepting accountability means that you recognize yourself and no one else as the final authority concerning what's best for you. Even given the fact that you must depend on others for certain things, and you may have little or no choice about other things, one thing is true: You freely choose what you enjoy, dislike, reject, tolerate, feel grateful for, or appreciate. If you are currently unhappy, you can decide to change that.

With new information come new thoughts. With new thoughts come new beliefs. New beliefs cause new behavior. That's how self-directed change works. That's how you get happy—by *choice, and not chance.*

In this chapter, you will learn more about Plato's take on the meaning and duration of pleasure. You will also hear what leading-edge research tells us about the "new science of happiness," as *Time* magazine dubbed it. When you've completed this chapter, you will:

- Know what Plato's four levels of happiness are and see how they differ from each other.

- Be familiar with some of the ideas coming from the science of happiness research.

- Understand that organizations as well as individuals can attempt to operate from a "Level Three" philosophy, even as they pursue profits.

- Realize what it means to be fully accountable for your life, and why accountability and lasting happiness are inseparable.

IF YOU'RE HAPPY, WE'RE HAPPY

Taken separately or together, the concepts in this book have one overriding purpose: To help you become happier. That's it. Everything else is secondary. Why is being happy so important? After all, happiness is just a pleasant feeling, right?

Wrong. The research is solid and the evidence is clear: Happy people laugh more, and laughter has stress-busting, healing properties. They make businesses more successful and profitable, relationships more harmonious, communities more desirable, and everything more fun. They also live longer. So what better reason could you possibly have for wanting to change something in your life? Achieving happiness is a worthy goal.

THERE'S HAPPY—AND THEN THERE'S *HAPPY!*

Make no mistake. The kind of happiness I am talking about isn't the fleeting pleasure that material things or brief sensual experiences create. It isn't a brand new car, or a beautiful pair of shoes, or a plate of homemade ravioli. It isn't the thrill of victory when you sink a difficult putt or beat your competition, either, although there's nothing wrong with any of these things. They are all great, as far as they go; we love them. The trouble is, those kinds of happiness don't go very deep or last very long.

Centuries ago, Plato taught that there are four kinds of happiness— some much more profound and longer lasting than others. Father Bob Spitzer, President of Gonzaga University in western Washington, introduced me to Plato's four levels of happiness more than ten years ago. Although it has been centuries since Plato thought and wrote about happiness, the value of his thoughts has not diminished. Understanding what he had to say is as important today as it was then, especially if you want to be happy in a lasting, deep-rooted way.

PLATO'S FOUR LEVELS OF HAPPINESS

1. **Level One Happiness** is all about immediate gratification. It is eating my mother's homemade ravioli. It is also a child at play, an addict getting a "fix," an adult driving a brand new car, or a couple sharing a kiss. It feels good and doesn't take much effort to generate, but it doesn't last long or satisfy us very deeply, either.

2. **Level Two Happiness** is ego-driven. At Level Two, we want to have more than…, perform better than…, or feel better than…someone else. We want this in order to feel proud of ourselves, bask in other people's approval, or experience a few moments of glory. Level Two happiness gives us those things—for a while. When I sink a basket when I'm up against much taller guys, the glee I feel is a perfect Level-Two moment. Or picture yourself beating a longtime rival at golf, or closing more sales than anyone else in the company, or winning a Best-in-Show ribbon for your dog or

painting. Like Level One, this level feels good, but only for a short time, and it is still all about me, me, me.

3. **Level Three Happiness.** As we grow older and continue to develop as human beings, most of us start to take less pleasure in material things, sensations, and ego gratification. As we mature beyond childhood and adolescence, we learn to postpone temporary pleasure to earn more permanent and meaningful happiness down the line.

   We stack up our experiences. We still enjoy that ravioli dinner and the new car, but temporary happiness doesn't motivate us as much as it once did. We still thrill at beating the competition, but it is not quite as satisfying as it used to be. We start looking for something more solid, deep rooted and dependable. That's what Level Three is all about. At this level, other peoples' happiness and well-being is very important to us. We want to reach out and help, to be of service, and to leave a lasting legacy. It is the deep, dependable, lasting happiness of Level Three that this book and Entelechy's education is all about.

4. **Level Four Happiness**. This is the deepest, most meaningful, and longest-lasting kind of happiness, because it is a product of our relationship with that which is eternal. Some spiritual/religious groups view this kind of joy as the ultimate goal. Some individuals see it in a uniquely personal context, while some don't think of it at all. Level Four is expressed as giving and receiving ultimate meaning, goodness, ideals or love. Level Four methods are always righteous, compassionate and patient.

THE NEW SCIENCE OF HAPPINESS

Until recently, modern psychologists and scientists weren't particularly interested in happiness. They studied pathology and neurosis, trying to understand why people weren't functioning optimally and what could be done about it. It didn't seem important, or it never occurred to them, to study happy people to see what was making them happy. Then, a few decades ago, the field of cognitive psychology was born. The connection between thoughts, emotion and behavior became a topic of great interest, so a great deal of important research was done.

Now, partly as a result of that research, many psychologists have begun to focus their attention in a more positive direction. They assert that happiness is not so much the result of genes, or luck, or even the absence of pathology.

In Part II, we'll look more closely at the new science of happiness and give you a snapshot of what positive psychology's researchers have discovered. I'll tell you what you really need to know and why you should care about this new science. I'll provide some pointers about how to use it in your own life. For now, though, I'll keep our focus on you.

ACCOUNTABILITY: HAPPINESS AND SUCCESS ARE CHOICES
Regardless of your individual circumstances, you have within you right now everything you need to achieve success and happiness. All you have to do is understand it and start using it. Although you may ask them for help or give them your heart, other people are peripheral. You and you alone are responsible for your own success and happiness, however you define them.

Success and happiness doesn't have to mean money, power or prestige. Scientists who study happiness tell us those things don't really figure into the equation at all. If it is going to have meaning and bring you a full measure of happiness, success must be defined by *you* and measured *on your own terms*. Unless complete accountability is part of your value system, you're almost guaranteed to fall short.

ALL OR NOTHING
What does "complete accountability" mean? Simply that you take responsibility for your entire life—all of it—the parts you like and the parts you don't like. It means the parts you want to keep because

they are working well, and the parts you dislike and intend to change. It includes the parts you are proud of, and the parts you'd prefer to hide. When you are completely accountable, you see yourself as you currently are, and you accept it. You also see yourself as you *want to be,* and you work to create it.

As CEO of "You, Inc.," you no longer let others decide what is best for you. You certainly consider other people's feelings, needs and desires, and you feel comfortable asking for opinions and advice. However, you are the one in charge of your life. You make the decisions.

CAUSES AND SOLUTIONS, NOT BLAME

You refuse to play guilt games. When things go wrong, you don't waste time blaming others for your own disappointments, worries and woes. Instead, you look for useful information and you ask constructive questions. What is really going on? Is there a more helpful, positive way to interpret the situation? What would I like to see happen here? What could I do to encourage that result? How might changing my own behavior change the outcome?

When you accept full accountability, you affirm that you are the primary causative power in your life, and you accept the responsibility that goes with it. You can't always control what happens to you, but you can control your response. Thoughtful response, as opposed to knee-jerk reaction, is a habit you can cultivate. If you are willing to train yourself to think and respond in ways that are more accountable and considered, you will find yourself feeling happier and more confident.

DENIAL DRAINS

No matter how much some people's lives may look like a bed of roses to you, they have problems and challenges. Everyone has them. When you accept complete accountability for your life, you grow from the challenges you accept and eventually master. Being accountable means shifting your energy from denial to acknowledgement, from criticizing and blaming to understanding, and to causes and finding solutions.

When you accept accountability, you become skilled at changing your focus from what's wrong to what *right* looks and feels like. You become skilled at developing clear mental pictures of what you want, and at setting the goals and planning the actions that will bring those pictures into reality. When you are perceived as highly accountable, you are also more likely to persuade others, and will earn their dedication and loyalty.

ACCOUNTABILITY EQUALS POWER: MAKE A PLAN AND FOLLOW IT

Now that you have become familiar with *The Ten Principles of Entelechy,* and how they can help you grow, why not decide to accept full accountability for your own happiness and success? *Choose to change,* instead of leaving change to chance. Why not start today?

1. **Set a goal.** The change you choose to start with should generate some internal excitement when you think about how it will feel to achieve it. You don't need to start with major change, either. Jim began with attractive, well manicured hands and moved on from there. Success breeds success, so it is usually wise to start with a smaller goal and work up to the big ones.

2. **Write an affirmation.** Describe the result of your goal in a one-sentence, first-person, present-tense affirmation. Describe how achieving this goal feels, as well as what it looks like. Write it down.

3. **Repeat and visualize your affirmation.** Ideally, every day. Some days you may want to affirm and visualize more often. No matter how often you do it, try not to be mechanical. Say the words and picture the outcome with genuine emotion!

4. **Track effort and record progress.** Keep your tracking system as simple as possible, but don't skip this step. If, after a few weeks, you're not getting the results you want, check the language you've used. Make sure it is generating real emotion. Check your surroundings, too. Distractions make it harder to focus and generate the mental pictures you are trying to internalize.

You might also want to form a weekly or bimonthly support group. Invite a few friends or colleagues who are serious about goal achievement to meet regularly, write and review affirmations, and offer each other feedback and support. Visit our web site, www.getoveritandgetonwithit. com, for more information about goal setting and using affirmations, individually or in groups.

Embracing accountability as a freely-made choice rather than something imposed on you is empowering. You create a wellspring of confidence tempered by humility that reaches into every aspect of your life. You generate the kind of lasting happiness that rests not in someone else's hands, but in your own—exactly where you want it to be.

REFLECTIVE QUESTIONS

1. When do I give up accountability, play victim, or try to blame others for problems at home? At work?

2. What makes me happy in a deep-down, lasting way?

3. What three goals could I set that would bring me more happiness? Write an affirmation for each.

Goal #1

Affirmation

Goal #2

Affirmation

Goal #3

Affirmation

樂

PART I REVIEW

In Part I, I introduced you to *The Ten Principles of Entelechy*, the foundation of Entelechy's educational process. These principles are both timeless and leading edge, and their purpose is simple: They help you understand your own thought processes and behavior, and give you tools that can be used to change them, if you choose.

Principle One, Take Change by the Hand, reflects the first law of life: The world in which we live is constantly and rapidly changing. For some people this is stressful; for others it is exciting. Which it is for you depends on your mental habits, attitudes and beliefs.

Principle Two, Open Your Eyes and Your Mind, explains that your reticular activating system is constantly scanning for information that is either threatening or valuable. When you open your mind to new ideas or set a new goal, your R.A.S. allows you to gain access to a world of useful information.

Principle Three, Understand How Your Mind Works, describes how you perceive and process information and make decisions. When you bring more consciousness to these mental functions, the benefits are enormous.

Principle Four, Adjust Your Explanatory Style discusses the differences between how optimists and pessimists interpret their environment and experiences. Optimism is an advantageous attitude that can be practiced and acquired.

Principle Five, Expanding Your Comfort Zone, talks about why you feel stress when you venture outside the familiar, which causes you to resist change. The better you are at avoiding stress, the less successful you will be at growth.

Principle Six, Exercise Your Imagination, explains that what you can do is limited largely by your ability to imagine it. The more clear and vivid your mental picture, the easier it is to make it real.

Principle Seven, Create and Resolve Dissonance, spells out how to create and harness the tremendous energy of cognitive dissonance to bring your boldest visions into reality.

Principle Eight, Say Yes to Your Future, is about how to create mental experiences that change your self-image in a very positive way. As a result, the kind of behavior you most want to see in yourself begins to feel natural and easy.

Principle Nine, Build Your Self-Esteem, reveals what self-esteem is, why it matters, and how it is developed. I outlined six practices that will work wonders for your self-esteem, if you bring them into your life on a daily basis.

Principle Ten, Accept Accountability and Get Happy, explains why accepting personal accountability is so vital to achieving happiness and success. When it is a freely made choice, being accountable empowers you. You become the final authority on what's best for you, and you understand that happiness rests, not in someone else's hands, but in your own.

PART II
APPLYING *THE TEN PRINCIPLES* OF ENTELECHY

USING *THE TEN PRINCIPLES* TO ENRICH YOUR PERSONAL LIFE

INTRODUCTION TO PART II
APPLYING THE TEN PRINCIPLES

Now it's time to accept accountability and put what you have learned to work. Knowing about *The Ten Principles of Entelechy*, but not applying them to your life is like knowing how to read but never cracking a book. Understanding without application doesn't do much good.

Part II gives you a wealth of ideas about how to apply *The Ten Principles* to your personal life, including health and fitness, and family and friends. It begins with The Balance Wheel, an exercise that provides a snapshot of where you are right now in several areas and helps you decide what you would like to change.

It's Up to You
Now that you have a basic grasp of how *The Ten Principles* work, you have 24/7 access to powerful techniques such as visualization and affirmation—practices that can help you deal more effectively with change and create more harmonious relationships. You can use these techniques and concepts to improve your creativity and energy, boost your productivity, and conquer many old fears. You can also use them to live in ways that create far less stress and much more happiness.

I hope that you are beginning to sense enormous new potential in yourself, and that you feel a new determination to bring that potential into reality. First, though, you must be willing to accept a new level of accountability, because no one else can create happiness and success for you. You have the ability, the tools and techniques. All you need now is the intention.

Before you begin Part II, set a clear intention. Approach the information with an open mind and a willing heart, and be clear about what you intend to get from it. Expect to find what you need to grow by leaps and bounds. Expect to waste no time chastising yourself for past mistakes. Expect to move forward, full speed ahead, into a better future. If your intentions are clear, your expectations are likely to be met and, indeed, surpassed.

Using *The Ten Principles* to Enrich Your Personal Life
The Balance Wheel Exercise

Your Big Picture

When you're growing where you want to grow, your life is working. The difficulty arises when you do too much "running on autopilot" and don't take time to assess what's really happening. If you are not spending time and energy on the things that are most important to you, it's important to be aware of it so you can correct it. The Balance Wheel exercise is designed to raise your awareness level.

Before going on to Part II, take a few minutes to complete this exercise. It will give you a clearer picture of what you value and will help you see how your time and energy are spent. It will also help you pinpoint areas of dissatisfaction and prepare you to use *The Ten Principles* in the most effective way possible.

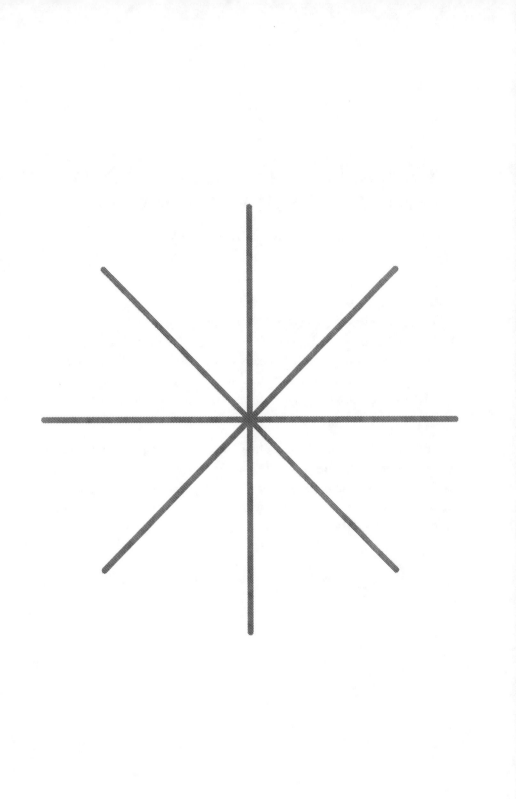

Instructions: The spokes on the wheel represent various aspects of your life. Label each with a descriptive word or phrase. For example: *family, career, health and fitness, spirituality, intellectual growth, social life, creativity/artistic expression, travel, etc.*

Make a colored dot on each spoke indicating the ***importance*** of that aspect. The center represents no importance (zero). The outermost point represents high importance (ten). So areas that are relatively important to you will have dots toward the outside; unimportant areas will have dots toward the center. When you have finished, connect the dots.

Go through the process again using a different color. Make a new dot on each spoke indicating the ***time and energy*** you are currently putting into this aspect. The center represents none, while the outermost point represents a great deal. Connect these dots with the second color.

Do this once more, using a third color. Make a dot on each spoke indicating the level of ***satisfaction*** you currently feel with this area. Connect these dots with the third color.

You should now have a pattern that looks something like a spider web. Look at the colored dots in relationship to each other and answer the following questions:

1. Where does your level of satisfaction closely match the value?

2. Where is value high but satisfaction low?

3. Where is value low but time and energy high?

4. Where is value high but time and energy low?

5. Do time and energy have any relationship to satisfaction?

6. Where are you not getting the results you want?

7. Are there areas where you would like to grow more or more quickly?

8. Are there other areas that you would like to make less important?

9. What have you learned about yourself?

10. What have you confirmed or brought into question?

11. Does this give you any ideas about goals you might set
    for the future?

If you're like most people, The Balance Wheel exercise made you more aware of the parts of your life you feel good about, as well as a few that you would like to change.

That's what this book and *The Ten Principles* are all about—making change an ally instead of an adversary. You can choose to change in ways that improve your satisfaction and success. You can choose changes that let you spend more time doing things that make you happy and less time feeling stuck or frustrated.

USING *THE TEN PRINCIPLES* TO ENRICH YOUR PERSONAL LIFE

VISION, VALUES, VIRTUES

IF YOU CAN'T SEE IT, HOW CAN YOU BE IT?

No matter what you call it—a sense of purpose, a mission, an ultimate destination, even desire— as a motivating, energizing force, nothing beats a vision. Its importance can't be overstated. With a clear vision, almost anything is possible. Without it, you may still do reasonably well, but your life will lack direction. You'll know that you could have been more, done more, and lived more fully.

That's because it is in our nature to grow. The entelechy in us requires it. How much we grow and in what direction depends on the quality of our vision. In other words, it's hard to get what you want if you don't know specifically what that is. While most people seem to know what they *don't* want, clearly and emphatically, they are much more likely to be vague about what they *do* want. They talk about wanting to be happy or content, have a good job, enjoy good health, a successful career, a good marriage, or have plenty of money. However, when asked for details, they hesitate.

After working with thousands of individuals and organizations, I know that the details matter. In fact, it is the spelling out of the details of a vision—making the vague concrete, the general specific, and the emotional payoff clear—that really empowers people.

Life rewards clarity. One of the reasons I made the affirmation and visualization process a key element of *The Ten Principles* education is that when you use it, you are speaking a primal language that brain and body understand—sensory, vivid and emotional. Messages transmitted in this language get through instantly, are retained, and have tremendous impact.

VALUES GIVE VISION MEANING

Naturally, you want that impact to be positive. Be sure the messages you send to the conscious and unconscious aspects of yourself are the ones you want to send—the ones that will generate the behaviors and feelings you desire—you need to be clear about your values. Values guide or qualify your personal conduct and interaction with others, as well as your involvement in a career. Like morals, they help you distinguish right from wrong and live in an integrated, meaningful way.

Values can pertain to many things. We can have values that relate to the environment, politics and politicians, finances and economics, art, sports, and so forth. Most of our values fit into three major categories.

1. Cultural and social values include ethnic diversity, religious faith, and tradition.

2. Professional values encompass things like industriousness, competition, recognition, and professionalism.

3. Personal values define you as an individual. They can and often do differ from those of your family, culture or workplace, and may include such qualities as honesty, helping others, creativity, independent thinking, challenge, feeling serene, having fun, being recognized, etc. The list is long.

Yet few people take the time or make the effort to get clear about what they value and why. If pressed, almost everyone will say they value honesty, integrity, kindness and the like. Further than that, they haven't usually given it much thought, and they have never tried to write any of it down. If you are serious about personal growth and want to make the most of your life, writing out your values and goals is a good idea. *Clear Values = Clear Vision = Purposeful Behavior.* Purposeful behavior is one of the keys to happiness and success.

FINDING YOUR MASTER VALUES

A virtue is a character trait perceived as good or worthwhile. Following is a list of virtues, by no means exhaustive. Read through the list. Then choose fifteen that are most important *to you*. Don't choose the ones you think *should* matter most to you. Choose those that really do.

acceptance	determination	idealism	responsibility
accountability	diligence	imagination	restraint
adventure	education	individualism	satisfaction
altruism	effort	independence	self-awareness
advancement	empathy	innocence	self-discipline
appreciation	endurance	integrity	self-interest
assertiveness	enthusiasm	intuition	self-reliance
autonomy	equality	inventiveness	self-respect
awareness	etiquette	justice	sensitivity
balance	excellence	kindness	service
beauty	fairness	love	sharing
spirituality	faith	loyalty	sincerity
calm	fantasy	mercy	self-esteem
care for others	fidelity	moderation	spirituality
charity	focus	manners	sympathy
curiosity	foresight	modesty	tact
cleanliness	forgiveness	morality	temperance
commitment	fortitude	nonviolence	tenacity
compassion	freedom	nurture	tolerance
confidence	free will	obedience	tradition
consciousness	friendship	openness	trust
continence	generosity	optimism	truth
co-operation	gentleness	patience	truthfulness
courage	happiness	perspective	understanding
courtesy	helpfulness	peace	unpretentious-
creativity	honesty	perfection	ness
critical think-	honor	perseverance	unselfishness
ing	hope	piety	utility
discipline	hospitality	potential	wealth
democracy	humility	prudence	well-being
dependability	humanism	purpose	wisdom
detachment	humor	respect	

Mission Possible

Now it gets harder. If you had to give up all but five of these virtues, which would you keep? These are your Master Values.

Record your Master Values here or on a separate sheet.

1.

2.

3.

4.

5.

Fortunately, you don't have to give up anything, but the exercise is valuable, nonetheless. Once you are clear about the values that drive and motivate you, creating a compelling, purpose-filled vision becomes easier. If your vision encompasses any or all of your five Master Values, transforming it into reality gets faster and easier, too.

It gets easier because when you achieve this clarity of vision and values, you feel like you have had your internal batteries charged! The power of a heart-centered, purpose-driven vision is amazing. After creating one, people come out of slumps, shake off pessimistic stances, take long looks at what they've been doing and saying, thinking and feeling, and decide to change. In the light of a shining, meaningful vision, everything becomes clear, and anything becomes possible.

In truth, it's always been possible. Now, however, *scotomas* have been busted. Reticular Activating Systems are on full alert, wasted energy is available, comfort zones are expanding, and the excitement is palpable. A value-driven, crystal clear vision is an incredible thing. If you have ever spent time around someone who has one, you've seen it. If you have one yourself, you will live it.

Finding Your Way

Without a clear vision, life is likely to disappoint you. What's worse, you'll disappoint yourself. You'll try this, try that, never feeling fully committed, and never really sure you're going in the right direction.

If you latch on to a vision other people create for you and you have never really owned it, or if your vision no longer fits the person you are, or doesn't reflect what you value, you won't fare much better. You'll find ways to become distracted, fail, sabotage yourself or wander off course.

What happens if you don't have a clear vision for your marriage or love relationship? No one can say with certainty, but a U.S. divorce rate of more than 50 percent tells us that marriage is tough enough as it is. Without a shared vision and values to keep you together, you are essentially stacking the deck against yourself.

No vision for your health and fitness? Good genes help, if you're lucky enough to have them, but don't bet your life on it. If lack of vision means you engage in unhealthy behavior, as it often does, here, too, you are asking for trouble.

In every area of life, lack of vision creates problems. Without it, how will you know whether your behavior supports or undermines success? How will you know when you're on track or off? If what you say you want in any area of life is so vague you can't describe it, how important can it be? How likely are you to persist when the going gets tough?

DESERVE OR DESIRE?

It is not uncommon to hear people talk about deserving to have this or that in life, or about not deserving it. Deserving something is not really the issue. We all have internalized ideals of our best or higher selves. Few of us consistently live up to those ideals. We may try, but as my father used to say, people are only human. We fail, we succeed, we veer off course, and we try again. Since we don't measure up to our own high standards, we may feel unworthy. As a result, on a subconscious level, we believe we don't deserve life's bounty. In subtle but serious ways that belief can sabotage us, time and again.

Forget deserve. Instead, think *desire*. What do you want? Why do you want it? If your purpose is aligned with your values, you're likely to find great satisfaction in working to achieve it. Even if your purpose serves only yourself, you still have a right to want it. Remember, developing a clear vision is not about what we "deserve." It's about achieving our heart's desire.

Trust your desires, but examine them. As you progress through various stages of maturity and growth, some of your values will probably change. Your desires will change along with them. There's nothing wrong with that. What you want to avoid are *unconscious* shifts—changes you're not aware of. In Principle Nine, the practice of living consciously is the first principle of building your own self-esteem. It's also the first practice, period. You can't be serious about your own growth without cultivating more consciousness of your own desires, values, beliefs and behavior. Denial and darkness limit us. Consciousness and light let us live fully.

GETTING SERIOUS

People who are serious about growth schedule a time-out every so often. They use the time to get clear about where they have been, where they are, and where they want to go. Following are several questions you can use to take a time-out of your own. Your answers will help you become clearer about your own values and vision.

VALUES & VISION WORKSHEET:
DATE:

THE PAST:
How have I spent my life thus far?

What have I accomplished?

If I had it to do over, what would I do differently? Why?

THE PRESENT:
How am I different now than ten years ago? Five years ago? One year ago?

What/who currently matters most to me?

If I were at the end of my life looking back, what about this time would stand out?

THE FUTURE:

What do I want to avoid?

What do I want to achieve?

What would I like people to say about me at my funeral?

GETTING REAL

Reality is what it is, no matter how much we would prefer it otherwise, or how much we protest. We need to be willing and able to see ourselves clearly. Never deceive yourself about what is or has been. Self-deception is the height of foolishness; self-awareness is the key to wisdom. If you can't see or admit what is really happening, how can you change it? If you don't see a problem, how can you resolve it?

Getting real about yourself and your life may mean experiencing some tension. You see yourself as you are, with all your problems, and you also see yourself as you'd like to be, problems solved. Whenever you hold two conflicting pictures in your mind, the result, as discussed in Principle Seven, is cognitive dissonance. Cognitive dissonance means tension and stress.

SELF-ACCEPTANCE AND CLARITY: CATALYSTS FOR CHANGE

The late Carl Rogers, founder of client-centered psychotherapy and respected author, said that when we accept ourselves just as we are, changing who we are becomes easier. Fred Rogers knew it, too, so he sent strong, steady self-acceptance messages to generations of kids through his award-winning public television show, *Mr. Rogers' Neighborhood.*

The positive relationship between self-acceptance and change is clear, for two principal reasons. First, it is easier to accomplish anything when you are not in an adversarial relationship with yourself. Carl Rogers didn't say we had to *like* what we saw in ourselves. He said we should acknowledge and accept it as true, for the time being. The truth may make you feel uncomfortable, but denying it will keep you stuck.

Second, as we've seen, allowing yourself to take an unflinching look at reality often generates cognitive dissonance—you see where you are. You know where you'd like to be, and you know your goal. They don't match. The result? Tension and stress. To reduce or eliminate that stress, you have two choices: You can change or deny your goal or you can change current reality. Whichever one you choose, consciously or unconsciously, depends in large part on which is clearer and most compelling—which carries the strongest emotional charge.

If your vision is indefinite and your values never clearly articulated, the vision will not hold up over time and its motivating force will be weak. Reality will eventually reduce it to a memory, one of those things you regret when you look back. If, on the other hand, your vision embodies and expresses your Master Values and heart's desire, it will be strong and inspiring.

Take the time to get clear about what you want and why you want it. Be clear about what you must do to get it and how you'll feel when that happens. Achieving this kind of clarity may take an hour, a few days or even longer. It is one of the best investments in time and in yourself you will ever make!

USING *THE TEN PRINCIPLES* TO ENRICH YOUR PERSONAL LIFE
HEALTH AND FITNESS

THINK HEALTHY!

It isn't news that our thoughts and emotions affect the health and well-being of our bodies. Exactly how this relationship plays out is still being discussed and discovered by scientists, but the fact that it exists is no longer in doubt. The repercussions have been nothing less than profound.

The health care establishment has some catch-up to do. In a field that is still guided, by and large, by outdated premises of Newtonian physics, the conventional wisdom says that your health is controlled by your genetic makeup. It also maintains that when things go wrong with the body, allopathic (traditional) medicine is the only kind that merits serious consideration.

Human beings often cling to false ideas with great tenacity, and scientists who pride themselves with being rational are no exception. For more than a decade, alternative therapies such as acupuncture, chiropractic and naturopathy have been gaining ground. Integrated medicine, embracing western as well as eastern methodologies and many approaches to wellness, are taught at major universities. The emerging science of *epigenetics* has forced many diehard traditionalists to sit up and listen.

Epigenetic means above genetic. Epigenetic research has shown that environmental influences, including nutrition, stress and other emotions, can modify genes without changing their basic blueprint.

The modifications can be passed on to future generations in much the same way as DNA blueprints are passed on via the Double Helix (Reik and Walter 2001; Surani 2001). If this is too technical, here's the bottom line: We are not prisoners of our genes—far from it. This is earth shaking news. At least it should be.

IF YOU CAN MAKE YOURSELF SICK...

It has long been known that we have the ability to make ourselves sick. There is abundant research showing that when we experience negative emotions—fear, hatred, panic, despair, frustration, rage, shame, guilt, and so forth—the brain produces powerful changes in our body chemistry. These changes set the stage for malfunction and illness.

Does this mean you should feel guilty if you become ill? Or, that you somehow caused it? Not at all. Guilt is a strong negative emotion, and it's the last thing you need to feel when trying to get well. At the same time, being accountable for your health and well-being is critically important. You need to understand the role genetics and lifestyle, including diet and exercise, play in creating illness and health. You also need to understand the role that thoughts and emotions, past and present, play.

As a child, you may have had experiences that set you up for the kind of health you now have as an adult. Did your parents speak of you as, "sickly," or "fragile," and did they treat you accordingly? Or, were you reminded that you were strong and resilient when you came down with an illness or broke a bone? Was illness seen as weakness, so you were expected to "tough it out?" Or, did you get extra sympathy and attention when you were sick or in pain? Were the people in your family and those around you strong and healthy? What stories did you hear about sickness while you were growing up? What health-affirming or health-eroding behaviors did you adopt as a result?

THE UP SIDE

A great deal of scientific evidence has recently accumulated to prove that it isn't only negative emotions that change body chemistry. Positive emotions do it, too. Love, laughter, hope, faith, compassion, joy, a sense of purpose, and feeling inspired—all have a significant effect on your body's chemistry and biological states. They strengthen the immune system, help produce specialist cells to fight disease, improve circulation and respiration, and lower stress. It is becoming widely accepted that in addition to making ourselves sick, we also have the ability to make ourselves well.

Dr. Andrew Weil, director of integrated medicine at the University of Arizona, well-known author and public television presenter, says, "Spontaneous healing is a common occurrence, not a rare event." (*Spontaneous Healing*, 1995) Our bodies are designed to repair and regenerate themselves. When we hear anecdotes about disappearing tumors and spontaneous remissions, we marvel. Yet no one thinks it strange when a cut or abrasion disappears over the course of a few days or weeks. Why have we conditioned ourselves to believe that the former is virtually impossible, but the latter is normal and natural? What might happen if we changed that belief?

Can beliefs really help create and heal disease? Can positive emotions make us live longer? How much is spontaneous healing like the placebo effect, or the result of self-fulfilling prophecy? After all, if you expect a certain outcome, you tend to do things that make that outcome more likely, whether consciously or not. How much spontaneous healing is simply biology? Can belief and biology be separated? Are they, like mind and body, different aspects of one system?

These are fascinating and vitally important questions that are the subject of ongoing research. We don't have all the answers yet. We may not have them any time soon. It is possible that the deepest mysteries of the body-mind connection may never be fully uncovered. However, we do know that the mind plays a major role in creating and maintaining the body's health and well-being. We know enough about how that interaction works to benefit from it, immediately and personally.

What Do You Tell Your Body? What Does It Tell You?
Your body communicates with you all the time. Pain is one of the most obvious communications—an unmistakable cry that something is wrong. Pain generally gets your attention quickly. But what about the more subtle messages of distress your body may be sending?

Fatigue, lethargy, high blood pressure, sleeplessness, shortness of breath, weight loss or gain, poor skin color, headaches, stomach or muscle aches—all are messages from your body. Do you give these less urgent communications your attention, as well? Or do you ignore them, hoping they will soon go away, or else respond quickly when you get around to applying a remedy?

Ignoring these signals sends a reply message to your body, "I don't care." If you would like to live in a state of vibrant good health, there are better ways to reply, and better strategies to employ. Becoming aware of your self-talk, whether it's aloud or in the form of thoughts, and learning to control it, is an important part of *The Ten Principles*. It's also an important part of taking charge of your life and your health.

What is your self-talk like regarding your own health and fitness? Do you believe that you usually catch everything that's going around? Or, are you positive you're healthy as a horse, so you don't even consider getting a flu shot? Do you get queasy just remembering something that made you sick as a kid? Or, do you smile at the memory, thinking how much things have changed? Do you avoid annual checkups because you feel fine and don't want to tempt fate? Or do you experience several unpleasant symptoms for which doctors can't identify a cause?

Remember, self-talk is incredibly powerful. For many years, one of my greatest fears was injections. No one enjoys them, of course, but most people learn to take them in stride. Not me. As a kid, I learned to hate and fear hypodermic needles to an extreme degree. I knew it. My friends knew it. Everyone in my family knew it, and if it ever seemed like I forgot, they reminded me.

AN "EXORCISM WITHOUT CLERGY

When *The Exorcist* first came out, I couldn't wait to see it. In the middle of the movie, though, I passed out. When I regained consciousness, all the lights in the theater were on, paramedics were at my side, an oxygen mask was on my face, and my feet were up in the air. It wasn't Linda Blair's head spinning around that sent me over the edge. It wasn't the green stuff spewing out of her mouth, either. It was the full-screen image of her getting an injection that meant lights out and a large coke all over my sister's lap! Had I known about *that* scene, I would have opted out. Similar embarrassing, needle-based episodes happened again and again over the years. It was a running joke to my brothers and sisters, but it wasn't funny to me.

Years later, as I was trying to invent reasons why I should skip a dental appointment because it usually meant a Novocain shot, I told myself enough was enough. I thought about how I had been conditioned to believe that this fear-based, panicky response was "normal," but was it really? I was certainly able to be calm in other stressful situations, and had no trouble coping with minor aches and pains—so the potential was there. All I had to do was change my belief.

That morning, I made a vow that old, negative conditioning would control me no longer. I created an affirmation to support that intention: *I breathe deeply and remain calm and relaxed when I get an injection.* I closed my eyes, spoke the words, and pictured it happening, in vivid sensory detail. I saw the needle, smelled the antiseptic, heard myself take a deep breath, imagined a brief sting, and felt the pride of accomplishment I knew I would feel when it was over.

It worked. I was elated that it worked so quickly and easily. I repeated the affirmation and visualization often enough so that, after a while, they weren't needed. Injections are no longer a problem. I use affirmations and visualization all the time to support my intentions for growth and change in virtually every area of life.

PERCEPTION, HOPE AND THE POWER OF INTENTION

In Principle Three, I discussed how your brain's Reticular Activating System helps you notice things that are either of value or a threat. I also emphasized the importance of keeping an open mind—exposing yourself to information and opinions that challenge your current beliefs. Whenever you lock onto a certain idea as, "The Truth," you may be locking out other ideas, and other truths that would benefit you.

If you care about promoting and protecting your health, why lock out anything? It makes sense to narrow your focus when you've done a reasonable amount of investigation and you're sure you know all you need to know or time is short. Maintaining a narrow focus can allow greater depth and help you feel secure. In the long run, however, wearing mental blinders is extremely risky. It assumes that nothing will change, that no new information will become available, and that the situation will remain static and stable. Those assumptions are foolish. Moreover, while a certain amount of risk is both necessary and beneficial in life, it's seldom if ever wise to risk your health. I *intend to be a healthy old man.*

Hope keeps us going and helps us heal. Despair makes persistence and eventual healing less likely. People who are seriously ill need as much hope as they can get to fight the good fight. Hoping or wishing for something implies that whether it happens is pretty much out of your control. Out of control is the last way you want to feel about your health. Intentions, on the other hand, are powerful and implicit acknowledgments that you are in charge.

All of your thoughts and feelings are forms of energy. Some, like fear and anger, are negative energy. They break down instead of build up, feel stressful rather than pleasant, and destroy or do harm. Hope carries a positive charge, feels good, and is constructive. Nevertheless, when you *intend* something, you boost the positive energy of hope with a turbo charge of accountability. You don't just hope health and fitness will happen. You make it your business to see that they do. You commit to doing whatever it takes.

CHANGE YOUR MIND, CHANGE YOUR BODY

In a *Discover* magazine interview, researcher/biochemist Nick Hall described a lecture he once gave. Since the audience was resistant to his ideas about the effects of mental and emotional states on immune system functioning, he believed he had to do something to get their attention. Otherwise, they'd just keep tuning him out. Therefore, Dr. Hall walked up to the podium, pulled out a copy of *Lady Chatterley's Lover,* and read them a particularly steamy passage. For a few seconds, everyone thought he had taken leave of his senses, but it did the trick. All eyes were on him when he asked the group, "If you're able to arouse your reproductive system with purely mental processes, why would you doubt that you do the same with your immune system?"

Now, more than a decade after Dr. Hall made his point in that lecture hall, the usefulness of visualization in illness prevention and treatment is widely accepted. Of course, everyone agrees that prevention is still the best long-term strategy for ensuring longevity and good health. Key questions for us all then become what's needed for effective prevention? What role should affirmation and visualization play, and where do we start?

CLARIFYING QUESTIONS, REALISTIC GOALS

What, exactly, do you want to change about your health and fitness? Why do you want those changes? No doubt you want to feel and look better, but in what ways? What will it take for you to look "better?" Can you see the details? What will feeling better be like, specifically? What's your long-term goal? What will it take to get there?

Ask yourself specific questions and write down your answers: What, who, when, where, how many, and how often? Pounds, cholesterol levels, blood pressure reading, belt size? Time at the gym, eat which foods, run how many miles? Eliminate what? What's desirable? What's merely okay? Do you want to go it alone or team up with someone? A good support system, workout partner or check-in group will boost the likelihood of achieving your goal. What about rewards and incentives? What happens if you lapse? How will you track progress? The more you know before you start and the more thoughtfully you plan, the better the results you are likely to achieve.

If you think you might need medical supervision, by all means get it before you begin. Whether you do it alone or in concert with a health or fitness professional, develop goals that are realistic for you—hard enough to be a challenge, but not so hard, you'll become discouraged and quit. Then make a specific plan, write it down, and follow it. Get feedback, from yourself and from others. Fine-tune the plan as you go.

The intention to be healthy and fit is a purpose that engenders well-being, body and soul. It will also generate energy—the energy of cognitive dissonance. Use it to fuel your mission. The behaviors that create and support health are not beyond you—no matter who you are or what your current state. It doesn't matter if you've tried before and failed, many times. What matters is whether you are willing to learn from experience. Tell yourself you were just warming up before. It's true, you know. Then get busy with the plan and start affirming and visualizing your new behaviors.

SAMPLE HEALTH AND FITNESS AFFIRMATIONS

- I love the feelings of vitality and energy I generate because I take good care of myself.

- It is easy for me to exercise every day because it feels so good.

- I love feeling strong, fit and healthy.

- I enjoy eating moderate amounts of healthful, nutritious food; it tastes great and I look and feel great!

- Good health is a choice I make every day of my life.

- I read labels on the food I buy in order to avoid saturated fat and empty calories.

- I am proud of the way my body looks and feels because I care about fitness and health.

- Exercising regularly makes me feel energetic and glad to be alive.

- Eating right and exercising gets easier for me all the time.

- I love being at my ideal weight and eating well-balanced, tasty meals.

USING *THE TEN PRINCIPLES* TO ENRICH YOUR PERSONAL LIFE

RELATIONSHIPS

HOW STRONG ARE YOUR CONNECTIONS?

Life is filled with relationships. Some mean more to us than others. Our connections and interactions with spouses/partners/sweethearts, children, parents and grandparents, siblings and close friends are considered primary. They have far more impact on us than those with colleagues, neighbors, distant relatives and acquaintances. Yet they all matter. Relationships have an enormous effect on our self-esteem, self-efficacy and self-image. They teach us to give and grow, love and laugh, and connect and create something larger than ourselves. It is within the context of important relationships that we do most of our growing. Few things matter more to your overall happiness than the quality of your relationships, especially those you value as primary.

The quality of your most important relationships reflects the quality of them all. If you are generally happy at home and have a good relationship with your family, your relationships at work and in your social life are probably running smoothly, too. If you have lots of conflict at home, it is likely you are having conflict on the job and elsewhere. If you are often angry or disappointed with your spouse or kids, you probably find yourself feeling the same way about quite a few of your co-workers, friends and neighbors. Funny how that works, isn't it?

Maybe it's not so funny. Actually, it makes perfect sense, because *your relationships won't get better until you do.* Unless and until you feel good about yourself and the way you're behaving, in your relationships and in the world, you won't feel good about the people you're relating to. Unless you accept accountability for your part in creating and maintaining the status quo, and until you decide to change *yourself,* nothing of substance in your relationships will change.

A BULL'S EYE VIEW OF YOUR RELATIONSHIPS

Take a few minutes to "map" the people in your life. In the center of the following bull's eye diagram, place a single dot to represent you. In the inner circle closest to that dot, write the names of your primary relationships. These are the people to whom you feel closest—usually spouse, sweetheart, children, parents, etc. In the next circle, add the names of those you care about but to whom you feel slightly less connected. Keep going until you have included everyone who matters. Place them closer in or farther out from the center, depending on how important the relationship is to you or how intimately connected to that person you feel.

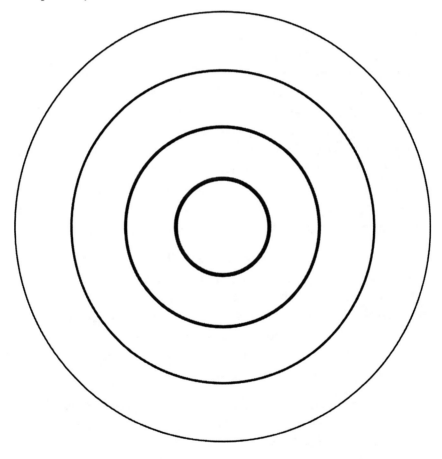

Now, on a scale of one to ten (ten equals great, one equals terrible), give each relationship a number to represent the *current* quality of that relationship. Be honest. No sugar coating.

WAKE UP AND BUST YOUR SCOTOMAS

For years, I figured I was just unlucky in love. I kept choosing women who made my life miserable. Time after time, things would look great at first, but after a few months or years, they'd turn sour. Bad would become worse. The details don't matter—it wasn't pretty. After two extremely traumatic and unpleasant divorces, I had learned two things. I knew exactly what I didn't want (more of the same), and I was absolutely certain my problem was not choosing the wrong women. The problem was ME.

Of course, it is possible to simply make poor choices, especially when you are young and inexperienced. Love, as they say, is blind, and reality is easy to distort to fit our fantasies. It was my belief about bad luck and choosing the wrong women that was making me blind.

In Principle Two, I introduced the concept of mental blind spots, or scotomas. When it came to relationships, I had so many scotomas for so many years, I was "scotomatose!" Gradually, I learned what I didn't want, but I still had no clear vision of what I *did* want. Being divorced forced me to wake up. I thank God for my children, because being a parent forced me to grow up.

THINK BIG, GROW INTO IT

Romantic love or even great sex isn't what makes long-term relationships thrive. Unrealistic notions about yourself or other people don't help you grow. You need to try to see the big picture of your life. What really matters over the long haul? What do you really want? What kind of climate do you want to create in your home, in your family, and all around you? What's your vision?

Take another look at the bull's eye you created a few minutes ago. Now that you have a fairly good idea of where your most important relationships are right now in terms of quality, it is time to start thinking about where, exactly, you'd like them to go.

By the time I met Darcy, the woman who I will live out my days with, I understood comfort zones, scotomas, and I knew how the R.A.S. works. I could explain how self-image drives behavior at the drop of a hat. I knew why affirmations and visualizations improve self-image and how the subconscious operates to resolve cognitive dissonance. I used this information all the time in my professional life, and I made a good living teaching it to others. It probably took as long as it did to apply these concepts to my love life, because I had locked on to the belief that I was some kind of romantic victim. When I busted that scotoma, I finally saw the truth. I wasn't a victim at all. On the contrary, I was fully accountable and very powerful!

So I stopped thinking about what I didn't want and started to try to get clear about what I did want in a relationship. Gradually, I created a Relationship Vision. I thought about what I brought to the past broken relationships that caused the relationships to fail. What was I responsible for? It wasn't just "those women" that caused it. Heck, I chose them. I thought about the qualities I most wanted in a life partner, and a mother for my kids, and I wrote them down—intelligence, sense of humor, integrity, energy, strong enough to be soft, soft enough to be sweet, and successful in her own realm. Mainly, I envisioned how it would feel when I knew for certain I had found her, whoever she was, and I described that in detail, as well as I could. I affirmed, in written and spoken language, meeting someone who had those qualities. I pictured it in my mind, though I admit I could never quite see her face. I even sang about it in my car!

Without a doubt, the most powerful thing I did during this time was work on developing in *myself* the qualities I wanted in this person. I wanted to be the kind of man that a talented, good natured, beautiful woman would hook up with, and I knew I couldn't fake it. I also knew it wouldn't be easy. Major change seldom is. It meant I would have to do a lot of work, but it is the kind of work that feels great when you get into it, so I was highly motivated. There were times when I wasn't sure it was doable. Maybe I was asking too much. Maybe I didn't "deserve" that much happiness. By then I knew enough to stop that kind of thinking. *The things you think about today create the things you'll experience tomorrow.*

QUESTIONS TO STIMULATE CHANGE
Imagine it is a year or two in the future. What would it feel like if your most important relationships were all harmonious, happy and

fulfilling? Hold that thought for a moment. Do any less positive thoughts start to bubble up? Do you begin telling yourself that such relationship happiness is impossible? If so, look deeper. What beliefs do you have—about yourself and other people—that stop you from trying for relationship happiness and harmony? How were those beliefs created in the first place? What affirmations and visualizations could you create that would help you alter those beliefs, and as a result, change your behavior? What else might you do to change your beliefs and behavior?

Try to answer these questions, even if it takes significant time. Write your answers down. Be unflinchingly honest. If you catch yourself lapsing into self-critical or self-pitying thoughts, reel yourself in. The purpose of your inquiry is to discover useful information, not to undermine yourself with needless guilt or negativity.

While you're at it, here are a few more questions to consider. What makes a relationship happy, as far as you're concerned? What, if it's rare or absent, makes a relationship unsatisfactory or even painful? What kind of person is easiest for you to like or love and what kind of person feels good to be around?

Easy to Like, Easy to Love

It's simple enough to teach to children, and powerful enough to transform lives. In general, the people who are easiest to like and love are those who:

1. **Help us feel good about ourselves.** They know what warms our heart, and they do it often. Whether it happens unconsciously or on purpose doesn't matter. Feeling unappreciated causes so much conflict, so many break-ups, so many disengaged employees, disillusioned spouses and depressed children! On the other hand, no matter how old we may be, when we feel genuinely appreciated and valued just as we are, it helps us to thrive and grow. You don't have to be in love with the other person to express appreciation. However, you do have to feel a basic sense of goodwill,

and the desire—the intention—to have a fulfilling, happiness-producing, mutually beneficial relationship.

2.   **Rarely criticize.** No one likes to feel that they are constantly being scrutinized by someone who has no compunctions about pointing flaws and weaknesses. This doesn't mean that we must accept everything about the other person in the relationship. It certainly doesn't mean that we should allow ourselves to be mistreated. If you don't already know this, it's time you did—*Criticizing people isn't the best way to get them to change.*

Think twice about criticizing anyone, especially a life partner, child, friend or family member. Just because you *can* doesn't mean you *should.* It doesn't matter whether you're "right," either. You are not an authority on how fast anyone else should grow and change, and you don't get to tell them what to do unless they are your kids. Even then, you don't get to tell them for long. People move in the direction of praise, but they avoid criticism and criticizers. Before you start dispensing criticism or unasked-for advice, make sure your intention is truly to help. Choose your words, tone of voice, and timing carefully. Aim for honesty *plus* kindness.

HIGH SELF-ESTEEM HELPS

The goal, again, is not so much to *find* these easy-to-like, easy-to-love people, but to *be* one. When you are, you will effortlessly attract similar others. If your self-esteem is shaky or low, you will constantly look to others for reassurance of your own value. Unfortunately, you will never get enough to convince you for long. You may even try to put other people down so you can feel superior. This happens often, and it amounts to dosing your relationship with poison. That's why I made "Strengthen Your Own Self-Esteem" one of *The Ten Principles of Entelechy.*

If you think you may have low self-esteem, review the six practices outlined in Principle Nine. Nothing can transform your relationships as profoundly as these practices, especially when combined with *The Ten Principles.*

BUILD A CLIMATE OF SAFETY AND TRUST

Among other things, intimacy means that you freely share private feelings—hopes, dreams, worries, fears, likes, dislikes, proud accomplishments, embarrassment, shame, and the unlovely facts about your clay feet. It means trust, coming and going.

You must do your utmost, even when you are angry or hurt, to make it safe for each other to tell and hear the truth. What makes it safe? Suspending judgments, criticisms and blame, and listening with one and only one goal: to understand.

Intimacy also means equity and equality. Both partners in a relationship need to feel that they are getting, on balance, roughly as much as they give—that neither one has a better deal. This usually doesn't happen automatically. It requires persistent effort, skill and time. Like successful businesses, successful relationships aren't easy. If you persist in doing the work, day after day, year after year, you will reach a point where it doesn't feel like work anymore. It just feels like what you do. It also feels like it's absolutely worth it. You do the work, and you get the rewards.

Both people in a relationship can learn how to create trust, build intimacy, listen with open hearts and share their thoughts and feelings with honesty and kindness. You can also learn to resolve conflict and talk to each other on a daily basis in ways that shore up rather than chip away at the relationship.

Here's a great place to start. Let go of the idea that if your partner would only change, everything would be fine. Then start thinking about yourself. *It's more important to be the right person than to be with the right person.* Just as I did, work on being the person you would like your partner to be. Set a good example. Do it to improve the relationship, because there's no doubt that it will. Do it for yourself, too.

Ten Thoughts That Can Transform a Relationship

1. Commit, not to the relationship, but to the *quality* of the relationship.

2. Redirect half of the energy you put into changing the other person to changing yourself, and magic will happen.

3. It doesn't do any good to know you have a bad attitude if you don't know how to change it.

4. When you know what you don't want, but not what you do want, you become fear-driven.

5. A relationship vision is a positive prophecy.

6. Relationships are like buildings—they need a strong foundation if they are to last. That foundation is compassion.

7. Unresolved conflict creates distance.

8. Authenticity is essential to intimacy. Intimacy means being seen and appreciated for our authentic selves.

9. If you want more connection in the present, let go of the past.

10. As long as the people in a relationship support each other to grow and evolve, the relationship will remain vibrant.

USING *THE TEN PRINCIPLES* TO ENRICH YOUR PERSONAL LIFE
ABUNDANCE THINKING

BEYOND POSITIVE

If you are a positive thinker, most of your mental energy is directed toward positive ends. You spend time thinking about how to improve your own character. You think about how to have better relationships. Developing your capabilities is important to you. So is giving to others. For the most part, you enjoy life. You believe the old saying, "Where there's a will, there's a way," so you look for opportunities instead of obstacles. You're not blind to potential problems, but you don't focus on them. You recognize your strengths and capitalize on them, and you don't waste time obsessing about your weaknesses. You tend to see other people through the same positive filters. You affirm what you want, work hard to get it, and believe the future is in your own hands. In short, positive thinkers are dedicated, hard-working optimists.

Abundance thinking is a fine-tuned form of positive thinking. It is built on a solid foundation of optimism and emphasizes profusion, plenty and gratitude. Abundance is the opposite of scarcity or lack. A belief system that embraces abundance generates prosperity. You gravitate toward joy and confidence rather than worry and stress. When you live, work, love, play and dream from a place of personal abundance, you cannot help but create more abundance. Love creates more love. Abundance creates more abundance.

Practicing Abundance

Repetition helps us acquire new beliefs and behaviors. It reinforces the neural pathways that facilitate ease and habit. The process of learning a new way to think or behave is in many ways similar to the process of learning to shoot baskets, read a profit and loss statement, or surgically remove an appendix. The best way to make an abundant mentality feel natural and the best way to make shooting a basketball feel natural are the same—practice.

Set a goal and make a plan. Then practice. Every day, try to see the world as a place of profusion and plenty. Every day, affirm that there is always enough of everything to go around. Every day, control your self-talk. Stop victim/scarcity scenarios. If you have seen life as a zero-sum game in the past, challenge that belief. If you have always figured that because some people have too much, others must go without, examine your logic. Start taking charge of your relationship to money, to abundance, and to success.

Right now, just briefly, imagine yourself as an abundance thinker. Imagine that the following statements about you are true:

- Whatever you desire is available in abundant quantity. You are clear about what you want, open to working for it, and prepared to use it wisely.

- If you need money, you will generate and receive it with gratitude.

- If you need people, you will find them or they will find you; the relationships will benefit everyone.

- If you need ideas, you will discover and grow from them.

- The more you give, the more you have to give.

- The more you sell, the more buyers there are.

- The more you know, the more you can teach and learn.

- The more you attempt, the more you will learn what works.

- The more you love and feel compassion, the more you will grow your ability to do and feel good.

How does it feel to affirm these ideas? What might happen if you visualized them, repeated them, and believed them, every day? Seeing is not believing; it's the other way around. If you don't believe, you're unlikely to see. If you do believe, signs of abundance will jump out at you—your reticular activating system in action. Instead of neediness and lack, you will begin to operate from a center of generosity and compassion. You won't have to pretend. You will be genuinely happy when friends and associates prosper. You will enter every transaction and relationship with your eyes wide open and a win-win attitude in mind. You will start expecting the best and behaving accordingly, in every aspect of life.

FIRST THINGS FIRST

If you want to change the way you experience abundance, the most important thing to change is your mind. Whether you develop it alone or with help, the first thing you need is a clear, fact-based picture of your current reality. Are you living beyond your means? Have you spent yourself into trouble? Is your dwelling or workplace crammed and cluttered with stuff you don't really need or use? Do the places you live and work reflect the self-image you want to have? Or do they reflect something you'd like to get away from? Do you over-consume, never feeling that you have enough? Have you developed a financial plan for your future, and a comfortable cushion in case of an interrupted income stream or other unforeseen obstacle? Is your retirement secure? How about your children's educations? Any investments? Obligations?

Once you have examined your current reality, you need a clear vision for the future and a reality-based plan that will get you there. The long-term goal is financial, emotional and spiritual abundance. Shorter-term, it may mean tearing up credit cards, selling things you don't need, or developing a budget. The sooner you have a plan to follow and the sooner you actually begin to follow it, the sooner you will be in charge of your own abundance.

Darcy and I come from working class families. Early in life we learned that people like us and our families had to struggle to get ahead. I am not sorry we were raised with a strong work ethic, but I wish we had learned more about how some of our beliefs handicapped us. I had to learn that not everyone who offered to help me in business was ethical. Darcy had to learn that she didn't have to do everything herself. We both had to learn how to articulate a clear, compelling shared vision and realize that success didn't have to mean a struggle. We could enjoy the ride more while in transit to our destination.

TURNING THOUGHTS INTO ACTION

To attract abundance, you must move from thought to action as soon as possible. We can think about abundance all we like, affirming and visualizing a relaxed, generous-spirited abundant life. But until we transform thoughts and words into action, not much will change. Here are five things you can do to create abundance:

1. **Become fiercely committed to your own growth.** Review your Balance Wheel. Create a clear, compelling Vision. Make a goal-achievement plan. (See #3 below.) Set up a reading, listening, and learning schedule; if you schedule these important things, they are more likely to happen. Research personal and professional growth. Listen to CDs, MP3s and tapes. Participate in seminars, trainings and other development programs. Get a coach or mentor. Start a success support group.

2. **Mentor others.** Teach what you know and be open to what others can teach you. If you have a talent for coaching kids, volunteer it. Help someone else grow. When other people benefit from your efforts and attention, you are putting abundance thinking into action.

3. **Create an achievement plan.** If you already have one, update it. Decide what goal-directed actions you will take

every day. Record them at day's end. Reward yourself at milestones. Celebrate major accomplishments in major ways. Adjust the plan when necessary. Be diligent, but try to make it fun.

4. **Visualize six abundance affirmations daily.** Write them on your calendar, screensaver, to-do list, Blackberry, PDA or journal. Put sticky notes in your car to occupy your mind at traffic lights. Stick them on the bathroom mirror and fridge. Don't let the words become routine. When you look at them, picture them. Feel them. Charge your visualization with emotional energy.

5. **Tap into the synergy of support.** Connect with others who share your interest in personal/professional development. Join or start a Ten Principles Abundance group. Meet regularly to support each other and share information. Log on to Entelechy's web site www. getoveritandgetonwithit.com, and join our Podcasts and blogs.

NEW THOUGHTS, NEW RESULTS: SEVEN ACTS OF ABUNDANCE

We draw many events, people and circumstances into our lives though the causative power of our thoughts and feelings. This isn't a mysterious process. It works on a simple principle—*When your mind changes, so does your behavior.*

As you begin to think differently about abundance, your behavior will begin to change automatically. Try to think about abundance in ways that will benefit you deeply and lastingly. Aim for the kind of "Level Three Happiness" discussed in Principle Ten. Our media-driven society urges us to desire and consume more and more, but if our sense of abundance depends on material things, our satisfaction will be shallow and short-lived. There will always be someone or something more desirable than what we have. High-level abundance thinking breeds contentment, not craving. It is fostered by these seven simple practices:

141

1. Give thanks every day.

Don't think about what you wish you had. Instead, take five minutes a day to remember what you do have. What's going well, though you may take it for granted? What's eased your load or given you a laugh? Take a step back and adopt the perspective of one whose troubles are far worse than yours. What would they envy? Write down your thoughts. Review them from time to time. Like generosity, gratitude greases the wheels of abundance.

2. Acknowledge and overcome addictions

Gambling, alcohol, drugs, food, shopping, spending, even seemingly harmless activities like Internet surfing, reading or working out can skid around the bend of moderation and become compulsive. Compulsions have a debilitating effect, eroding self-respect and sapping energy. But even though the body and mind may be powerfully attached to a substance or activity, the spirit is always free. If you are addicted to something, use your spirit to free the rest of you, and get help. Abundance thinking isn't likely to happen inside a mind preoccupied with satisfying addictive cravings.

3. Remember what lasts

The most lasting happiness comes from using your talents to serve a purpose greater than your individual pleasure. That kind of happiness doesn't depend on how well you are doing with your goal achievement list, whether you are driving your dream car, or living in your dream house, enjoying perfect health, or cruising at the top of your profession. It is a choice that has nothing to do with what you have and everything to do with who you are.

4. Be generous

A materially rich, spiritually empty life heightens fear and insecurity. To assuage these unpleasant feelings, our culture bombards us with messages telling us to acquire even more material goods. In our drive to acquire, we can become wasteful, contemptuous of those who have less or envious of the affluent. Abundance thinking calls for a different kind of consciousness. It means we must learn to tell "want" from "need," be thoughtful consumers, and experience abundance in ways that reflect our personal values.

5. Simplify

The more we need in order to be happy, the more difficult happiness is to achieve. Needing less is a surefire way to make sure our needs are more easily met. Acquiring fewer things mean fewer choices must be made about their acquisition, maintenance and protection. A simpler lifestyle means more time and space for personal enrichment and less stress. Simplifying can lead to an increased sense of security, too, if it is your decision to pare down rather than have something forced on you. What's more, simplicity is often simply beautiful. Every day for a week, pick one superfluous thing, practice or belief to discard. See how good you can get at it.

6. Give generously

Abundance flows where generosity goes. The more you give, the more you will benefit. In what areas do you presently hold back from giving? That's where your abundance flow is blocked. You can open it. If you want more love, give love; if you want more money, give money; if you want more wisdom, offer your own; if you want happiness, make other people smile.

7. Keep cravings in check

Overindulging in anything, even something you love, leads to discomfort and discontent. If you forget your goals to indulge cravings more than occasionally, you will probably sacrifice long-term success for short-term pleasure. Even if you could string a lifetime of pleasing sensations together, each new one would have to be more pleasing than the last, or a sense of dissatisfaction would plague you. On the other hand, whenever you feel blessed by what you have and able to treasure simple pleasures, you are living in the heart of abundance.

Using *The Ten Principles* to Enrich Your Personal Life

Accountability

What Accountability Is and Is Not

The word *accountable* is derived from an ancient Roman term that meant, "to stand up and be counted." We hear it often these days, but it can mean different things to different people. For our purposes, accountability is much the same as answerability, responsibility, and other words associated with the expectation of an account-giving. Who expects this account? Your boss does, if you have one. So does your family, most likely, and your community. No doubt your spouse or sweetheart expects you to account for your behavior. Your church may expect it, too. Certainly your government does, in many important respects.

When you are fully accountable, it is *you* who expects the accounting. You care enough about your own character to consciously monitor yourself. Silently or aloud, you ask yourself, "What am I thinking? What am I doing? What's going on around me? How do I want to respond?" Accountability itself is a kind of consciousness. To be accountable, you must be aware of and willing to accept the consequences of your own choices, and your own actions.

Occasionally, when you talk to people about accountability, things can get a bit tense. Some people reject the idea that they have 100 percent accountability for their lives. Maybe they have been struggling with a serious illness or were injured in an automobile accident. Perhaps their spouse or sweetheart left them without warning. Maybe they have been assaulted, robbed or cheated by a business partner. They feel like victims. "Are you telling me I'm to blame for what's happened to me?" they may ask. "Do you want me to believe I should feel accountable?"

No Denial, No Blame, No Victims

Being accountable doesn't mean taking blame. The kind of accountability I am talking about has nothing to do with blaming yourself or anyone else. No matter how much you might like to believe otherwise, you can't control everything that happens to you. No one can. There are two important things you, and all of us, *can* do:

- Look at the possibility that you played a part in creating the situation. Did you make a habit of taking good care of yourself? Were you tuned in, and paying attention? Did you take risks you shouldn't have avoided, or did you fail to safeguard something? Were you lazy about trusting someone who hadn't earned your trust? Did you stand by and do nothing when you should have spoken up or intervened? Were there warning signs you ignored?

  The purpose of these questions is information gathering so you can do things differently in the future. The purpose is not to provoke guilt or shame. Resist any temptation to use your answers as reason to heap blame upon yourself. Just don't go there.

- Remind yourself that how you respond to unpleasantness, difficulty or even tragedy is in large part up to you. You can use what's happened as an excuse to feel angry, bitter, defeated, hopeless, and helpless. You can use them as justification for self-sabotage, staying stuck, and giving up. Or, you can use adversity to learn from and grow.

When you see yourself as a nonentity, victim or pawn, you lose power, energy, and self-respect. When you choose to be accountable for everything in your life, and stop blaming others for your problems, you become more powerful. When you refuse to be victimized, ever, and decide to use everything that happens as a catalyst for your own growth, you stand tall in your own life.

WHO'S AT THE CONTROLS?

Simple survival requires us to possess many skills. The pursuit of dreams requires many more. In other times, people had to learn any number of skills just to survive. Today, most of us specialize in a single discipline, trade or craft, and work at honing our skills throughout much of our lives. We outsource much of the rest. As a result, we may feel a bit uncomfortable at the helm of our own existence. We question our ability to make wise decisions when it comes to things outside our expertise, so we give away accountability. We let others decide how we should safeguard our health, raise our children, spend our money and leisure time, decorate our homes, look and behave, feel and respond. When things go wrong, we blame others and feel victimized.

When you blame someone else for a problem in your life, you sidestep the real issue and reveal your own abdication of power. The authority to take ultimate accountability for your life is simply a matter of believing that you have the resources and intelligence to cope with any circumstance life sends. As with self-esteem, building confidence and self-efficacy is a matter of knowing what practices work and following them. If you need help, help is out there. The authority figure in your life should be you.

BECOMING YOUR OWN AUTHORITY

All of us want to look good to other people. We want them to like us, think well of us, approve of who we are and what we do. Sometimes, though, our desire to please others and gain their approval can become a problem. It can prevent us from taking the accountability we need to take to be powerful people.

When you are usually trying to put yourself in the best possible light and feel anxious about provoking someone else's disapproval, it's a problem. When you will not make a decision or even a move without finding out what others think, it's a problem. When you suppress your own desires and yearnings because they may not meet with someone else's approval, it's a problem.

There is simply no way to be your true self without creating some disapproval. Someone, sometime, somewhere is not going to like something about you. So what? That doesn't mean you're a bad person. In fact, it doesn't say anything at all about you. Whatever it says is entirely about the person who disapproves.

If you are usually pretending to be different so that people will like or approve of you, you will know you're a phony. The cognitive dissonance and stress you create with that kind of deception is enormous. What's more, if you're always trying to control what other people think of you, you'll be seen as self-absorbed and insecure, no matter how hard you try to mask it with a veneer of nonchalance or confidence.

It takes courage to be yourself—without conceit, but also without apology. Do you believe so strongly in the person you are that you refuse to pretend? Do you accept yourself, with all your shortcomings, and expect others to do the same? Do you allow others to be who they are, too, without judging them as defective, inadequate or foolish? One of the surest signs of low self-esteem is constantly putting others down, finding them incompetent, inadequate or unworthy of respect. That goes double when you run yourself down.

POP QUIZ #1

How much accountability do you currently demonstrate in the following important areas?

1 = little or none and 5 = 100 percent

____	Doing what I need to do to ensure my physical health
____	Doing what I need to do to ensure my emotional health
____	Doing what I need to do to ensure my financial security
____	Doing what I need to do to be a lifelong learner
____	Doing what I need to do to ensure harmonious relationships
____	Doing what I need to do to succeed in my career/ job
____	Controlling overeating, drinking, shopping, gambling, and drug use, etc.
____	Controlling workaholism and preventing burnout
____	Avoiding rescuing and unhealthy dependence of others
____	Managing my time; having time for everything that matters to me
____	Managing stress, overcoming fear
____	Taking the necessary steps to live a balanced, fulfilling life

Try writing and visualizing affirmations for areas in which you scored 3 or less.

Pop Quiz #2

If you have trouble accepting full personal accountability for your life, answering these questions may offer insights. After you have pinpointed your trouble spots, write and visualize affirmations to address them.

- How easy it is to believe that you alone determine your life's direction?

- How often do you blame others for where you are today?

- How easily do you admit mistakes, to yourself and others?

- How easy is it to believe that you can control your responses when negative events occur?

- How easy is it to depend solely on yourself for acceptance, affirmation and approval?

- How willing are you to be accountable for the strength of your self-esteem?

- How often do you feel sorry for yourself or "beat yourself up?"

- How easily can you let go of guilt when you fail to rescue others?

- How successfully have you practiced self-affirmation?

- How successfully have you practiced anger control and "letting go?"

People who fail to accept accountability for themselves often become self-pitying, depressed, chronically angry, dependent, despondent, pessimistic, stuck, fearful, obstinate, hostile, aggressive, passive, insecure, obsessed, or just plain lost.

Their accountable counterparts tend to go through life feeling confident, powerful, willing to risk, authentic, resilient, open minded, and optimistic. The choice is yours.

Using *The Ten Principles* to Enrich Your Personal Life
Resiliency

Adversity and Opportunity

All of us have to deal with obstacles and setbacks in life. Occasionally, we even have to deal with tragedy. No one is exempt—not movie stars, millionaires or world leaders, no matter how picture-perfect their lives may seem to others. How we deal with adversity is critically important. Obstacles stop many people in their tracks, causing confusion and frustration, and thwarting achievement. Setbacks can be springboards to success, if you have plenty of resiliency to help you bounce back.

Your environment doesn't have to dictate your feelings. Realizing this and acting accordingly will help you become more resilient. What usually happens when you let what's going on around you determine how you feel? When things go well, you feel great—happy, optimistic, energetic, and positive. When something goes wrong, you're in trouble. If it's something important that's wrong—a key relationship dissolves or you lose your job, you may come unglued. You feel like a victim— helpless and hopeless. Your mood turns angry, resentful, or apathetic and depressed. You give up control over your life.

Instead of choosing to be a victim or getting angry, which is really just another expression of victimhood, you can choose to take charge of how you respond. When you get right down to it, the only thing in life you can control is what goes on inside your mind. To exercise that control, though, you have to *decide* to do it and *learn* how. It doesn't happen automatically.

When you decide to take charge of your thoughts, and your self-talk, you become very powerful. Even so, you may still feel disappointed when things go wrong. If they are important things, you may even feel discouraged or disheartened for a while. However, you can choose to use adversities as opportunities to learn and grow. You can improve your ability to bounce back when you hit a rough spot and build the mental toughness that comes from meeting the challenge of adversity. You can minimize your own down time.

No More Fear of Failure

In Principle Seven, I talked about cognitive dissonance—the tension caused by trying to hold two different ideas about reality in your mind at the same time. In times of adversity, it is the dissonance between your expectations and your current reality that gives you so much grief. Your expectations may include the unspoken, and unrealistic belief that adversities shouldn't happen to you. They occur in other people's lives, of course, but when they knock on your door, you think something's wrong. You don't want to admit that they are inevitable, or that you secretly fear them.

Obstacles, setbacks and the feelings that may accompany them are nothing to fear. It is far better to acknowledge them than to deny them. Some self-help books imply that if you can just get good enough at positive thinking, you'll avoid problems and heartache, but they are misleading. Moreover, life's problems serve a purpose. When we look back on the troubles we went through, and the obstacles we stood up to, most of us can see that they taught us valuable life lessons.

How can you learn to be a good problem-solver if you never have problems? How can you develop strength of character if you never struggle with difficulties? How can you feel compassion if you have never felt pain? How can you fully understand the satisfaction of success if you have never experienced frustration and failure?

This does not mean that you should feel grateful for adversity or see it as a great gift. Mastering the art of resilience can do much more than restore you to the place you were before adversity struck. It can enable you to come out of the experience changed for the better.

YOUR RESILIENCY RESUME

To improve your resiliency, start by taking inventory. Think back over your life. List every time you can recall when you felt like giving up, but didn't. List every disappointment you recovered from, every failure you learned from, and every setback you eventually managed to overcome. These questions can help you recall:

- What "failures" in my past, including childhood and adolescence, turned out to be blessings in disguise?

- What difficulties have helped shape my character for the better?

- What hurdles in my relationships have motivated me to grow?

- When did I feel like quitting but kept going? What did I learn?

- What seemed like a mistake at the time, but turned out to be a good thing?

Your answers should help you see that you already have a wealth of resiliency experience. If you are not impressed, look more closely at your self-talk. You may be minimizing your accomplishments, and thinking things like, "Everybody does this stuff; it's no big deal." If so, stop. Get real. In the first place, you're wrong—everybody doesn't do them. In the second place, why would you want to devalue yourself like that?

Choose another, more positive point of view, such as, "Wow! Look at all the times when I've turned setbacks into comebacks, held on when I felt like letting go, learned from my mistakes, and grown as a person." If you believe in giving credit where credit is due, don't leave yourself out of the equation. Positive self-talk is important all the time, but never more important than when dealing with adversity.

GETTING BACK ON THE HORSE

A few years ago, when someone I trusted embezzled a large amount of capital from our company, it was so unexpected and demoralizing, I

153

almost threw in the towel. Looking back, I don't know what I would have done without family and friends. I knew that if I stayed down too long, being down would become the norm. Therefore, I used the principles. As a result, the company is stronger today than ever, and those dark days are barely a memory.

In light of a painful fall, getting back on the horse can feel like a big risk. The longer you play it safe, the greater the weight your disappointment takes on. The longer you postpone taking action, the harder it can be to start moving. A good support system can be extremely helpful. Find a mentor who can advise you or hire a personal coach. Create a clear mental vision of the end-result you want. Affirm and visualize that vision, and inspire yourself with stories of others who have succeeded in spite of major obstacles.

It's important to realize that after a shakeup, you will probably need to do some things differently—things you may never have done before—and you will probably have to stretch your comfort zones a bit, too. That means you can expect to feel some tension and stress. Again, the important thing is not that you experience stress, but how you choose to respond.

Affirm and visualize calm progress. Decide to interpret some of the stress as excitement—a sign that you are venturing into new territory. Other good stress reducers include aerobic exercise, meditation, prayer, yoga, or anything else that absorbs your attention and makes time fly. For you, maybe that means pulling weeds or reading a good mystery. For me, it's shooting hoops, boating with my kids, or cooking an Italian dinner. Remind yourself that living a totally stress-free, risk-free, and completely comfortable life means living without growth.

When adversity strikes or you're reeling from an unexpected obstacle, it is impossible to overemphasize the importance of surrounding yourself with people who believe in you. They will help you reaffirm your ability to recover from setbacks, grow into your goals, and eventually succeed. Avoid those well-meaning folks who urge you to give up when times get tough. When your own self-talk becomes doubtful or negative, you need strong, encouraging, credible voices to counteract it. Wherever they are, whether across the table or across the room, on TV or on CDs and tapes, find those voices and listen to them.

Using *The Ten Principles* to Enrich Your Personal Life
Effective Goal-Setting

Why and How to Set Goals

Hundreds of studies have proven that setting clear, specific, and challenging goals results in higher performance than setting no goals, or goals that are vague and hard to measure. Consequently, savvy goal-setters have a distinct advantage over the rest of us. If you want to accomplish more, set more goals—but do it right. Do it systematically.

Start by making sure that each goal you set has the following characteristics:

- **It must be specific.** Instead of saying, "I will exercise as often as I can," a specific goal would read like this, "I will jog for at least thirty minutes, four times a week, on the treadmill at the gym in foul weather, or outdoors in my neighborhood when it's fair." A specific goal should define:

WHO will be doing the behavior—usually you;
WHAT the behavior will be;
WHEN it will occur; and
WHERE it will occur.

- **It must be challenging, but attainable**, neither too easy nor too difficult. Don't try to move mountains, at least not at first. Don't set yourself up for a walk in the

park, either. You are the best judge of what represents a
stretch for you. Aim for that feeling.

If this is your first time trying a goal-setting system, here's a good way to
start. Practice using it to establish or strengthen these three important
habits. Reinforcing them will help you with every goal you set in the
future.

1. Repeating and visualizing affirmations

2. Increasing positive self-talk

3. Decreasing negative self-talk

Following the guidelines for specificity and degree of difficulty above,
try writing a goal statement for each.

GOAL #1. REPEATING AND VISUALIZING AFFIRMATIONS

GOAL #2. INCREASING POSITIVE SELF-TALK

GOAL #3. DECREASING NEGATIVE SELF-TALK

Check your goal statements by answering these questions: *Can the
goal be measured as it is currently written?* If not, rewrite it so that the
behavior you want is countable. *Does the goal clearly define WHO,
WHAT, WHEN, and WHERE?* If not, spell it out. *Does the goal represent
a "stretch," but not so much that it seems unrealistic?* If not, revise it. Aim
for realistic yet challenging goals.

OVERCOMING OBSTACLES

When we try to change our behavior, we often find that our "default settings" pull us back to our old ways of doing things—even if the old ways weren't working well. Relapse can feel frustrating, but if we anticipate obstacles, we can develop strategies to overcome them. In many studies of self-directed behavioral change, people who had a plan for how to deal with obstacles did much better than those with no plan.

Review your three goal statements. List some things that might prevent you from making your best effort. Include your own thoughts and feelings, if appropriate, as well as things you'd describe as circumstantial. After you've identified potential obstacles, think of several things you could do to overcome each, and list them.

GOAL #1: REPEATING AND VISUALIZING AFFIRMATIONS
What obstacles might prevent me from achieving this goal?

1.

2.

3.

What could I do to overcome them? (List several for each.)

Obstacle 1

Obstacle 2

Obstacle 3

GOAL #2: INCREASING POSITIVE SELF-TALK
What obstacles might prevent me from achieving this goal?

1.

2.

3.

What could I do to overcome them? (List several for each.)

Obstacle 1

Obstacle 2

Obstacle 3

GOAL #3: DECREASING NEGATIVE SELF-TALK
What obstacles might prevent me from achieving this goal?

1.

2.

3.

What could I do to overcome them? (List several for each.)

Obstacle 1

Obstacle 2

Obstacle 3

TRACKING AND REWARDING

Tracking your progress is a key part of the process. "What gets measured, gets done" is an old saying from the business world, but it's true in your personal life, as well. In this case, measuring involves: 1) recording your goal-directed behaviors, and 2) identifying what helps or hinders. Your recording system should be simple and easy to use. Ideally, goal-directed behavior should be recorded as soon as possible after it occurs. If that's not possible, do it at the end of each day. Jot down:

- What you did well

- How you might have done better

- What helped or hindered

Rewards are important. The best time for a reward is after an initial effort, at significant goal milestones, and when the end-result has been achieved. The best kinds of rewards are those that grow along with your accomplishments. Choose things that give you real pleasure; don't choose a massage unless getting one is a special treat. Rewards should also come in the form of positive self-talk. Reinforce your efforts and achievements with lots of congratulatory words and thoughts. Go ahead, brag a little. You have a right to feel proud of yourself!

SPEAKING OF SUPPORT

Feeling accountable to others as well as to yourself can increase your level of commitment and improve your likelihood of success. External support can come from many people and places, but specialized goal-achievement support groups (Weight Watchers, etc.) are known for their effectiveness.

Why not organize a group yourself? Round up a few others who like the idea and get together once a week for eight to ten weeks. Keep meetings short—no longer than an hour. Three group activities that have been shown to be important in promoting successful change include:

1) sharing experiences, 2) modeling (learning from the way others succeed or cope with obstacles), and 3) coaching each other. Build your group around them, and see how well it works for you.

Written contracts can be powerful ways to support goal achievement. They facilitate focus and clarity; can be consulted often, and most importantly, inspire greater commitment. If you're serious about goal achievement, create a written agreement. It should include your goals and the behaviors involved for achieving them, how you intend to track progress, the rewards you will receive and when, and a concluding statement indicating that you agree to abide by the contract's conditions.

Signing the contract sends a strong message to yourself. It says, in effect, "I take this seriously. I am fully committed to following this plan and to putting forth my best effort. I intend to see this through to success."

Using *The Ten Principles* to Enrich Your Personal Life
Maintaining Momentum

Use It Or Lose It

"Use it or lose it" is as true for what you have learned from this book and *The Ten Principles of Entelechy* as it is for brain power, muscle strength, and cardiovascular health. If you don't use *The Ten Principles,* fail to practice affirming and visualizing your goals, refuse to stretch your comfort zones and expand your own accountability, you will eventually lose motivation and momentum.

What can you do to make sure this doesn't happen? There are several things you can do to virtually guarantee it.

- **Schedule regular time alone** to reflect, recharge, and examine your goals. Too many of us leave this to chance. Then, because most of us are so busy these days, it never happens. Some people complain that it's hard to arrange solo time. They say the only time they spend alone is in their car or the bathroom! That's all the more reason to schedule this time. Put it on your calendar, with your other important appointments, and plan to retire to a place where you can be undisturbed. Perhaps that's a table at Starbucks, or an easy chair at a bookstore or a park bench. Aim for one hour, once a week.

- **Review and visualize your affirmations.** Set aside between five and fifteen minutes at least once, preferably twice a day. Visualization and affirmation are powerful processes—if you use them.

- **Keep your entelechy alive**. Review what you have read in these pages and any notes you have taken. Read other books that expand on *The Ten Principles* or explore related ideas. Investigate Entelechy's web site and see what supporting materials you can find. Start or join a discussion group and share success stories. Discover other products and services that will help keep you energized, focused and optimistic.

- **Increase positive self-talk, decrease negative self-talk, and keep a rubber band handy.** If you look for what's wrong—for the flaws and imperfections—you will find them. If you look for the positive, the beneficial, and the praiseworthy, you will find them. Of course, knowing you have negative thoughts is one thing; stopping them is another. Awareness is the key. You can't stop negative thoughts that you don't know you have.

  Here's an idea that can help you gain awareness and control of negative thoughts. Wear a rubber band around your wrist. The next time you catch yourself with a negative thought, snap it and say, "Stop!" If the thought comes back, do it again. You don't need to hurt yourself; just a little reminder pinch will do. Then substitute a positive affirmation for the negative thought. If you catch yourself thinking, "I can't stand that person," snap the rubber band and say something compassionate and kind, such as, "I look for the good in everyone." If you find yourself complaining, and say, "I'll never learn to do this," give the band a snap. Then tell yourself a more useful truth, such as, "I am proud of my ability to learn whatever I choose."

- **Build your own self-esteem.** Principle Nine is about building your self-esteem through six life-changing practices. If you do as they suggest, you will go a long way toward maintaining your momentum. It is worth noting that in the process, you must often question the values and beliefs that were handed to you when you were young. If some don't serve you well, or if they cause you to feel inadequate or unworthy, it will strengthen your self-esteem to put more affirming, positive beliefs in their place.

You must also work to keep your promises, whether to others or to yourself. Every time you fail to keep your word, a piece of self-respect is chipped away. When that keeps happening, it doesn't matter how much of a good a front you put on—you are in trouble. You must be as good as your word, and your word should be as good as gold.

- **Become fit and stay that way.** People who exercise regularly feel better about themselves, sleep more restfully, enjoy better health—especially as they get older—and have better sex lives. If that isn't enough to make you put on your Nikes, how about this: People who exercise regularly accomplish more. It's true; a great many studies bear it out. Mental and physical energy are directly linked. Exercise energizes. Optimists are not couch potatoes! Regular aerobic activity is important to both physical and mental health.

- **Practice patience and persistence.** Your ability to be patient with yourself *while you persist* is crucial. You are growing into your goals. While leaps of growth are great, and they sometimes happen, most growth takes place in increments. Aim for persistent effort and gradual progress. If progress seems stalled or if you find yourself drifting away from your goals, it may be time to review your vision. Does it still motivate you? Is it still something you truly want?

If so, learn from the lapse and resume your efforts. Remind yourself why you are doing what you're doing in the first place. Remember what persisting through the hard parts will bring you. If your vision no longer moves and motivates you, ask yourself what needs to change—you or the vision? The kind of life you live depends on your habits, attitudes, and beliefs. It really is that simple. Change what you think about, and your life will reflect the change.

How's your momentum mojo?

1. What do I believe is preventing me from spending regular time alone to reflect on my goals, evaluate progress and strengthen my commitment? What message am I sending to myself when I fail to do this? How could I overcome these obstacles? Am I willing to experiment by scheduling solo time for the next thirty days?

2. On a scale of one to ten (ten equals perfect), how diligent have I been at writing, repeating and visualizing my affirmations? What would it take to bring this number up to a nine or ten? Am I willing to do what it takes?

3. What could I do to help keep *The Ten Principles of Entelechy* alive in my life?

4. Where/when am I most likely to entertain negative thoughts? What might I do to avoid this in the future?

5. In what areas could my self-esteem use strengthening? What could I do to build it?

6. On a scale of one to ten (ten equals perfect), how do I rate my physical fitness? What excuses do I give myself to avoid exercise? How do I feel when I am at my best, physically? Could I develop a plan to steadily improve my strength, flexibility and cardiovascular health? What might I do to ensure that I *follow* the plan?

Using *The Ten Principles* to Enrich Your Personal Life

Personal Affirmations

The following affirmations reinforce the material in Part II. Use them as written or as guides for writing your own. Visualize and *feel* what you describe. Believe in the truth of the statement, and repeat the process often.

- I feel centered and energized because my life is well balanced.

- Affirming and visualizing my goals energizes and motivates me.

- Decisions are easy for me because I am clear about what I value and why.

- I always have time for the things that matter most to me.

- I take good care of my body because it makes me feel strong and energetic.

- I enjoy eating moderate amounts of delicious, nutritious food.

- My relationships keep getting better because I keep getting better.

- My relationships thrive because I am a patient, considerate, and loving person.

- The more I give, the more I have to give, and the more grateful I feel.

- I am happily in charge of my life and completely accountable for my behavior.

- I bounce back quickly from setbacks and learn from my mistakes.

- I have all the inner resources I need to rise to any challenge.

- I am excited by setting big goals and I patiently persist in achieving them.

- I feel optimistic because I have a plan for my future and I follow it.

- I know where I'm going because I often review my goals and track progress.

- I am worthy of success and happiness.

- I grow in the direction of my thoughts, so I love thinking positively.

- Everything that happens to me is an opportunity to learn and grow.

PART III
USING *THE TEN PRINCIPLES* IN YOUR PROFESSIONAL LIFE

USING *THE TEN PRINCIPLES* IN YOUR PROFESSIONAL LIFE
CULTURING SUCCESS

WHAT'S IN A CULTURE?

Just as your personality is the sum of your thoughts, feelings and behaviors, culture is the unique personality or character of an organization, including its values and beliefs, policies and procedures, ethical standards and rules of behavior. Culture sums up "how things are done around here." It guides the people inside the organization as to how they think, behave and feel.

The values that create culture permeate our working lives. Whether we work for ourselves or for someone else, whether it is a large or small company, a local or international nonprofit, a hands-on or hands-off operation, we care about our experience while we are there. We care about such things as:

- The hours we work each day and each week

- Whether our workplace is fun, stressful, or something in between

- How decisions are made and communicated; knowing what's going on

- How co-workers interact; how employees and management interact; the degree of competition and cooperation between individuals and departments

- Flextime and/or telecommuting

- Whether we work alone or in teams

- Whether we work under heavy or light supervision

- Whether we have a clear path to advance within the organization

- Whether our efforts and accomplishments are noticed and appreciated

- The physical environment, including offices and cubicles, common areas, rules regarding office space, use of MP3 players, headphones, etc.

- The "norm" for what people wear—casual days, always casual, or dressed to the nines?

- Whether education is provided, both to hone job skills and keep us positioned for promotions or future jobs

- The quantity and quality of perks (break rooms, gyms/play rooms, daycare, parking, etc.) and other benefits (credit unions, vacation and sick leave, retirement savings, profit sharing, bonuses, incentives, etc.)

- How much time outside the office we're expected to spend with co-workers

GETTING IT RIGHT

Some corporate cultures are highly competitive and adversarial, while others are highly cooperative and synergistic. Some are growth avoidant, while others seek growth like plants seek light. Some cultures are adaptive; they value people and processes that create positive change. Others are un-adaptive; they are self-absorbed and risk-aversive, valuing order and conformity.

A few standout organizational leaders manage to get it right. They have or are in the process of developing a clear, compelling vision of what is possible for them and their people. That vision has been shaped by experience, fueled by desire, strengthened by setbacks and sustained by patience. I have had the pleasure of working with many gifted leaders, such as, Dennis Clements at Lexus, Jim Hagan at Fieldstone Mortgage, Bill Heard, Bobby Cremins, Leyla Vokhshoori at Nordstrom, Rafa Ballesteros of Banco Santander, Steven Smythe with Mercedes Benz and the list goes on, who seldom think in terms of either/or. Their companies value people, processes and profits. What's more, they value the environment, their communities, and even their competitors. These leaders intend to create and sustain a culture where good people can feel proud to contribute their efforts. They are not willing to leave "how it is" at their companies to chance. They are committed to creating an environment, in their personal and professional lives, that supports their vision and values. As Dennis Clements put it years ago, "Build a culture where your people have pride in the organization and enthusiasm for its works."

WHAT'S IT LIKE WHERE YOU WORK?

What's the culture in your company? If you're an organizational leader, do you know what it's like in the trenches? If you think you do, how do you know? From whom do you get your information? How do they know? Could there be reasons why they might not want to tell you the truth or "sugar coat" it? After talking with thousands of people in hundreds of organizations, I have learned that the people at the top—the ones who make the big decisions—are often mistaken when it comes to describing their organization's culture. However, the people carrying out those decisions know exactly what is happening and will be glad to tell you, if they believe you really care.

If you were asked to escort a stranger around your organization and he or she asked you the following questions, how would you answer? Would your responses change if you were writing them in a private journal, talking to your spouse, or your best friend?

- What five words would you use to describe your company?

- What is it like to work there? Do you enjoy it?

- What is important to your company?

- How are employees valued? How do you know?

173

- What skills and characteristics does the company prize?

- Do you know what's expected of you?

- How do people from different departments interact?

- Are there opportunities for training and education?

- How are people promoted?

- What behaviors are rewarded or celebrated?

During the course of a lifetime, many of us will spend more time at work than with our spouses or children. If you want to be happy, successful and productive, find work inside an organization where your personality meshes well with the culture—a place where you have a voice, are respected for who you are, and have opportunities to grow. If you are an organizational leader, do whatever it takes to create that kind of work experience for your people.

CREATING A POSITIVE CULTURE
Here are four steps leaders and managers can take to create and sustain a proactive, and positive organizational culture.

1. **Honor the past**
   Understanding the organization's history can help foster an important sense of identity and belonging. Tell stories about the company's founders and notable past accomplishments. Tell positive stories about the present, as well, and link them to the past, thereby creating an exciting sense of a shared future.

2. **Think and speak unity**
   Leaders who are skilled at bringing people together use the words "we" and "us" a great deal. With the goal of creating a sense of unity and *esprit de corps*, design work assignments that encourage teamwork. Discuss organizational challenges in ways that make them

everyone's concern. Publicly applaud and reward team rather than individual accomplishments.

3. **Show people they are valued**

Train managers to help people manage their careers by showing a genuine interest in their growth and development. When people are hired, initiate them in ways that show concern for their well-being. When senior managers take part in orientations and training programs by speaking personally to new recruits, it sends a powerful message. Throughout every aspect of training and development, stress the value of the organization's culture and people.

4. **Increase contact and communication**

Help people in different departments or divisions stay in touch. This is particularly important in large organizations, but it matters in every case. Arrange conferences and meetings so that people have time to socialize. Bring people together for picnics, parties and other special events. Work to create inter-group collaboration. Cross-train or move people laterally so they can spread ideas and better understand the big picture.

USING *THE TEN PRINCIPLES* IN YOUR PROFESSIONAL LIFE
THE BIG THREE: VISION, MISSION, AND VALUES

DRIVEN BY ENTELECHY

If someone were to ask, "What drives you?" there are many answers you might give. Perhaps you would say that your driving motivation is a desire to succeed in your career or to be part of a happy family. Maybe you would say that you are driven by a spiritual purpose—to serve God, other people, or your community. Perhaps you are driven to earn enough money to buy a new home, put your kids through college, or build a nest egg for your retirement. No matter what answer you came up with, or even if you found it hard to be specific, you would probably be aware that something inside you is moving you toward growth.

Centuries ago, Aristotle identified this internal force that drives human beings toward self-development and fulfillment. He called it entelechy. All of us have it. We are born with it. If we let it—if we acknowledge it, respect it, and put it to good use—it gives us the drive and energy to do whatever it is we want to do.

In the movie, *The Pursuit of Happiness*, the main character, Chris Gardner played by Will Smith, made a choice not to be the kind of father his was. Instead, he made the positive choice to be a loving, and caring father to his son. He did not choose the path of least resistance which would have been easy during the times when he was struggling and homeless. He chose the road less traveled. He was driven by that force to pursue happiness.

You, too, have a choice. You can elect to tap into this powerful energy, using it to help you grow and be more than you ever thought possible. Or, you can turn away from it, keeping yourself small, becoming lazy and complacent instead of challenging yourself to grow.

The wonderful thing about entelechy is that the more attention you give it, and the more you believe in it, the more powerful it becomes. As you consistently acknowledge and tap into it, you become ever more masterful at using your own internal energy to undertake and accomplish progressively bigger things.

AWARENESS + DESIRE + ACTION

Tapping into your entelechy involves a combination of awareness and desire, followed necessarily by action.

Awareness. You remind yourself that the power to control your own growth and shape your own life is within you. You can't always control your circumstances, but you can choose your response to those circumstances. How you respond will heighten or diminish your awareness, and boost or reduce your growth and sense of purpose.

Desire. You get very clear about exactly what it is you want to have happen. In other words, you create a vision for yourself and a goal or set of goals, based on your awareness and desire.

Action. You make a plan and hold yourself accountable for doing what it takes to achieve your goal, believing all the while in your own power to bring about the desired results.

DISCOVERING YOUR PURPOSE

Many people seem committed to professional endeavors that they never consciously chose or planned to pursue. They more or less drifted into their careers or jobs, and they seem to think that the shape of their lives is a result of circumstance. They are not motivated by a vision and have no sense of mission other than "keep those paychecks coming." Needless to say, many of these people find their working lives boring, unrewarding or exhausting.

One of the premises upon which I have based *The Ten Principles of Entelechy* is that each of us has been blessed with a purpose, although almost no one is born with an understanding of its scope—that needs to be discovered or uncovered. If you feel directionless—as if you, too, have drifted into the work you do—striving to discover your purpose can help you realize your true potential. It will help you live a more authentic, productive, and satisfying life.

Discovering your purpose is not always easy, even though some lucky people feel a kind of "calling" that makes it simply a matter of listening and following. Most of us have to expend a bit of effort to excavate our authentic selves and sense of purpose. We may try out different types of work, consult career counselors, work with coaches and mentors, and question ourselves relentlessly until we feel we have found our niche. Ideally, your life's work will encompass activities that allow you to express your intelligence and creativity, live in harmony with your values, and experience the basic pleasure of simply being yourself.

WHY BE MISSION DRIVEN?

This question comes up often in the work we do. The answer is simple: so you never lose sight of your greater purpose. Whether you are an individual or an organization without an unwavering focus on mission and vision, it is easy to become bogged down in the day-to-day routine. Without mission and vision, both business and life can feel purposeless and boring.

Vision statements and mission statements can be power-packed drivers in a company culture when they are done right, and when they are used to release the entelechy of the people inside the organization. The best missions and visions are catalysts. The worst are carefully crafted, but too long and overly detailed. They are often framed and prominently displayed, but they are too much to memorize and remember—often too much to bother with at all. Almost no one pays attention to them. Almost no one lives them. If you took them down and substituted famous quotations or excerpts from eloquent speeches, no one would notice, because none of the real people in the organization talk like that.

Ideally, an organizational mission or vision statement does not describe the obvious. Instead, it embodies the exceptional and extraordinary. Most of all, it should be four things: true, clear, succinct and exciting. It should also answer four questions:

1. How do we make a positive difference, each and every day?

2. Why is it that the world can't possibly get along without the work we do?

3. What are we most proud of?

4. Why are we so special?

The best business mission and vision statements often use un-business-like words, such as beauty, caring, service, and even soul. They express the organization's values and purpose, often unconventionally, and always stirringly.

MISSION? VISION? WHAT'S THE DIFFERENCE?

Some companies don't bother to distinguish between mission and vision. They may have a separate values statement, but if you question people in the organization about their vision and mission, they'll give the same answer for both. So what is the difference between mission and vision?

As simply as I can say it, your mission is what you do best every day, and your vision is what the future looks like because you do it so exceedingly well. To help differentiate between them, you might compare them to another old debate: management versus leadership.

- **For mission**: think managing with greatness and untamed strength, while improving everything daily.

- **For vision**: think leading with inspiration and courage; seeing the future in terms of possibility, and embracing the challenge of change.

A mission bolsters the confidence of an organization by influencing its ever-present self-talk, such as, "We do this, and we are the ones who should be doing it, because we are arguably the best at it." Mission provokes revolutionary ideas about the mundane, banishing mediocrity.

Vision creates a momentum of growing anticipation about the future. Change is embraced as a step closer to that compelling picture of what's coming next. Excitement about the future dominates any apprehension about the uncertain. Change is recognized as the catalytic converter it truly is.

Turn mission and vision statements into mantras that people can actually say, while beaming with pride. "This is my company, and I'm glad it is" is the feeling they evoke—a feeling you can see in everyone's eyes. Both mission and vision should be alive; both evolving, reinventing, and growing as the organization and its people grow.

Tear down that tired old plaque on the wall. No one reads it and you don't need it. Trumpet the clarion voices of mission and vision instead.

USING *THE TEN PRINCIPLES* IN YOUR PROFESSIONAL LIFE
FINDING YOUR BALANCE

THE CRUNCH

These days, nearly 50 percent of American families have two wage earners, while fewer than 20 percent are "traditional" breadwinner and homemaker pairs. Add to that the facts that job security is a thing of the past, raising kids seems tougher today than ever before, and marriage is still an enterprise that, even when it's going well, demands a great deal of time and energy. The result? Balancing complex work and family roles is a constant, draining source of stress for many of us.

Psychologists tell us that stress comes from two primary sources—role strain and spillover. *Role strain* happens when the responsibilities of one role interfere with performing others. For example, a job that requires exceedingly long hours or a great deal of travel negatively affects the way we function as a spouse or parent. When conditions and relationships in one area of our lives affect another area, it's called *spillover*. Constantly changing work schedules, a hypercritical manager or a high-pressure office can disrupt family life. Likewise, family problems can have a negative impact on the job.

Here are four things you can do to help minimize stress and develop a better sense of balanced living:

- Clarify and prioritize values

- Set value-driven goals, and adjust your expectations

- Actively manage time

- Understand control and learn to let go

CLARIFY AND PRIORITIZE VALUES

If balancing work and family demands is important to you, take time to examine your values. Most of us are aware of a few of them, but sometimes important values remain unconscious or unarticulated. We don't question or even acknowledge many of our values until we have to take on a new role, or until we find ourselves feeling conflicted. It sounds harmless, until you realize that if you have unconscious values, it increases internal dissonance. When you get clear about your values, you will have taken the first step to shutting down stress.

Some values may be at odds with each other. For a while, I believed that it was important to arrive early at my office, before most other people. I also believed it was important to leave a tidy, clean kitchen behind me at home. As a result, I was in trouble five days a week. When something unexpected happened and everything took longer then usual, my tension level would skyrocket. Ballistic kitchen cleaning almost always results in more mess than clean. It didn't take long before it was clear that I needed to sit down and have a serious talk with myself. I needed to get in touch with my values again, to see if they'd changed, and think about how they were interacting. I tried to see where those values came from and whether they were helping me achieve my goals. After doing this, I decided that it was time to modify some of them a bit in order to ease the unproductive stress and strain.

Try it yourself if you have felt a tension-producing work-family conflict. When it comes to family roles, the places where strong but conflicting values are likely to show up generally center around the big three issues of money, religion, and child raising. They may also include housework, meal preparation, meal times, third-party child care, car and house maintenance, quality and quantity of couple/family time, education, and entertainment. Take a look at these things and get clear about *why* you're doing what you're doing. What are the values behind your behavior? See if you can turn them into complete sentences. Write them down.

Set Value-Driven Goals, and Adjust Your Expectations

Goals help define how you use your time. When values are the foundation of your goals, they can create major motivation—amazing infusions of energy. If you have too many or poorly prioritized goals, the opposite happens. You can blow your stress circuit breakers trying to be too many people or do too many things, particularly when all are of equal or near equal importance.

To reduce role strain, consider putting some goals on hold. You might want to modify some, and perhaps even let go of a few altogether. You won't know what makes sense until you are clear about your values and priorities. What matters? What matters *most?*

Perception is not part of the problem. Perception *is* the problem. Your expectations about the way things should be and the way people should behave are often harder to identify than your goals. Attitudes and expectations that don't serve you well today can create an overload of stress.

If you have unrealistically high expectations about being everything to everybody, performing all of your roles well all the time, or being "perfect" in any way, perhaps it is time to reconsider. While it defaces the amiable Clark Kent stereotype, it is nevertheless true. In real life, the so-called supermen and superwomen of the world are often exhausted, irritable, or angry. They are tough to be around and even tougher to be.

If that sounds uncomfortably familiar, try adjusting your attitude and expectations. It's a bit like adjusting the monitor on your computer. Once you know how to do it, things look instantly better. Let go of expectations that are unrealistic or no longer support you. Upgrade hard-and-fast needs to preferences. Write and visualize affirmations for new and improved expectations that will make your life easier and happier.

ACTIVELY MANAGE YOUR TIME

Managing a job or career, running a household, finding time for family and friends, involvement in social or community events, continuing personal growth, and planning solo time to reflect and recharge are areas that demand your time. These may not sound so terribly difficult just reading about them, however, trying to do all of them day-in and day-out, year after year is another matter.

Surveys have shown that after completing all the have-to's in a typical day, many of us have, at most, one to two hours of discretionary time. Even when we are reasonably efficient, that's a big time crunch. We may find ourselves doing things right, but not doing the right things. How often do you plan and schedule specific activities that will move you toward your goals? What about when the goals are neither concrete nor pressing? For example, if your goal is to improve your relationship with your son but there is no motivating crisis, you are less likely to make a plan detailing how you intend to improve things. That's because relationships are complex day-to-day processes. Without crisis to motivate us, we may find it difficult to identify activities that will work to improve them.

It may help to ask these questions:

- What are my expectations, for myself and for others?

- Where did these expectations come from? Are they realistic?

- Do they help or hinder me in reaching important goals?

- Am I balancing concrete/material goals with relational/people goals?

- How will I know when I have reached my goals?

- What do I need to do today to move myself toward them?

Learn To Let Go

What does it means to you to be "in control?" Do you believe that you have more control if you do everything yourself? If that sounds like you, you probably already know that your attitude is stopping you from reaching many of your goals; others it simply slows down.

Learning to delegate can be an enormous help. If done correctly, delegation can turbocharge your ability to get things done and achieve your most important goals. When you think about making changes in this area, particularly about behaving differently, you may find yourself face-to-face with your values about what should be done and how. Don't be surprised if you encounter some inner resistance when you try to reallocate home or work tasks. Several old beliefs may surface, but try to let reason rule. Let go of your old ways of doing things if they no longer serve or support you. Don't forget, though, that the emotional satisfaction we derive from some tasks and the power attached to certain responsibilities are important aspects of the division of labor. In other words, holding on to tasks that build your sense of self-efficacy and self-esteem generally makes good sense.

Careful planning and plenty of communication should always be central to change efforts that involve others. Here are some specific ideas that can help you plan and achieve better personal-professional balance:

- Hold family meetings. Make them fun as well as useful.

- Schedule time *regularly* for concrete and relational goals.

- Be flexible. Revise plans when they don't work. Don't sweat the small stuff.

- Understand what you can control (the six inches between your ears) and what you can't (everything else).

- Develop a sense of humor or grow the one you have. If you can keep each other laughing, you will probably be fine.

- Remember that, like you, the balancing process is continually evolving.

Using *The Ten Principles* in Your Professional Life
Coaching That Works and Mentoring That Matters

Why Coach?

It's a fast-moving, dog-eat-dog world, right? Coaching takes work. It takes a certain amount of commitment, too. It eats up time, if you're serious about it. So why should you spend your precious time and energy trying to teach someone else what you already know? Let them figure it out for themselves or let someone else do it. With life as busy as it is, who has time for that kind of thing, except pros who get paid? We have heard those words or similar words many times, but the people who say them are almost always young, inexperienced, or both. They are also missing out.

It is one of the greatest pleasures on earth to watch another human being grow as a result of something you did or said. Many studies and surveys report that most people feel that way. Level Three living is what makes us happiest in the long run, and with the exception of a few coaches who do it for the money or to stroke their own egos, coaching is a Level Three activity.

Not that the coach doesn't benefit, which I will say more about in a moment. When you coach or mentor another person or group of people, your purpose is clear and simple—you want to help them in a meaningful way. Obviously, then, coaching is a good deal for the person being coached. They get to learn the ropes from someone who knows, short-cutting their journey to competence, and perhaps even to mastery. They get support and guidance as they grow.

The coach gets something, too. It feels good, which is reason enough, but it also enhances self-esteem, increases self-awareness, and gives you a chance to express what psychologist Erik Erikson called generativity. Generativity is the desire to give back, to leave a legacy—something that becomes important to many of us in our later years. Another perk that many people who coach others get is a kind of energy exchange. The coach gives out wisdom and gets back an increase of his or her own creativity. Coaching can revitalize you to an amazing degree. It recharges your batteries.

THE CHALLENGE OF COACHING

The best coaches see more in us than we are able to see in ourselves. Their vision is clearer because they can see not only who we are, but also who we could be. They see our potential. Even though they are committed to helping us be and do our best, coaches are not gods. We have seen high-level professional coaches behave in ways that are hardly laudable. We have watched well-meaning coaches berate and belittle those they were coaching, hoping to goad them into a performance spike. We have seen all kinds of counterproductive histrionics and profanity in the name of coaching, in conference rooms as well as locker rooms. We have seen coaches who wanted to control everything and coaches who were afraid to touch the reins.

Maybe we haven't seen it all, but I have been involved in various kinds of coaching for most of my adult life—working with everyone from little kids to basketball stars to business leaders—and I have coached using *The Ten Principles* for more than a decade. I have read many studies and even more books, thought about it a great deal, and I've come to a few conclusions. Here, in a nutshell, and in no particular order, is what I have learned about being a good coach, inside an organization or inside a gym:

- Praise effort and achievement, but never flatter.

- Be clear about expectations and ground rules, but allow for the unexpected.

- Be patient, but not lax.

- See those you coach in terms of their potential and help them to see it, too.

- Tell the truth; don't sugar coat, but don't be brutal, either.

- Don't under- or overestimate the competition.

- Listen and observe as much as you talk.

- Don't get angry.

- Soft-peddle weaknesses, and capitalize on strengths.

- Do what you say you will do and expect it in return, but make room in your philosophy for human frailty. Give everyone a break now and then.

- Recognize deficiencies and compensate for them.

- Be an example of what you would like to see in those you coach.

- Pay attention—100 percent. The closer you get to 100 percent, the less you have to think about what to do and the more you'll just do it. It's called flow. When you are in it, you are completely engaged. On the playing field, it's when you have game. On the job, it's when time flies. It's fun.

You do need to have fun. If it feels like a trip to the dentist, you will want to stop doing it. So, last but far from least, bring some lightheartedness to the coaching experience. We love to learn from people who make us laugh.

COACHING FROM A TEN PRINCIPLES, LEVEL THREE POSITION

The Ten Principles education can't possibly contain everything you need to know about how to achieve goals, succeed in your endeavors and grow—but it goes a long way toward covering the fundamentals, and it offers a great place to jump off from. That's why, whether I am coaching managers and executives or basketball players, whether I'm doing it one-on-one or in a group, or whether they're adults or kids, I use The *Ten Principles* as a foundation. No matter who I am coaching, they talk about:

- The importance of clarifying values and purpose

- Self-talk and self-image—how they are formed and how they control behavior

- How to stretch comfort zones, put the reticular activating system to good use, and take advantage of cognitive dissonance

- What self-esteem and self-efficacy are and how to build them in others as well as in yourself

- How to develop resiliency so you can learn from mistakes and turn setbacks into springboards

- How affirming and visualizing change works to facilitate change

- How high-performance people think and behave

- What it means to become goal- and action-oriented

- How to think in terms of the greater good instead of your personal agenda

- The advantages of a self-management program that works

- How beliefs, habits and expectations shape behavior, and how behavior enhances or undermines whatever game you are playing, whether you are a corporate leader or an underdog competitor, a working mom or single dad, a top exec or this week's temp.

Everything on this list is a concept in *The Ten Principles*. Separately and together, they can address virtually any coaching issue that comes up. If you are lucky enough to have a coach who knows these principles well, or to be one of those coaches yourself, you know how they can facilitate dynamic, positive change. As our contractor friend says, having *The Ten Principles* is like having a workshop full of precision tools instead of just a hammer and saw; there are no limits to what you can build.

The Ten Principles help people get clear about what they want and then actually "build" it. As you saw in Part I, they offer a flexible, relevant, proven-effective process that merges timeless wisdom with leading-edge science and bona fide experience. Whether you are a coach or you have one, whether you want to help your team process more loans or score more goals, sell more cars or create happier customers, bring what you've learned from these pages and *The Ten Principles* to the table. Coach using this information and you will be amazed by the positive change it generates.

In addition to challenging others, good coaching challenges us to walk our talk, and to teach by example. Whether we like it or not, we will be scrutinized by those we coach, and whenever we take on coaching responsibilities, our credibility and integrity are on the line. We want to measure up. We want to honor our own high standards. Of course, coaching tends to attract people who care about growth and development; so many top coaches also coach themselves and have their own coaches/mentors.

MENTORS RULE

Coaching is a lot like mentoring, but there's a shade of difference. Mentoring means a kind of "taking under your wing" and guiding, while coaching is often more task, skill, or goal specific. Whatever you want to call it, the experience of having a mentor is something we highly recommend. I have had many, for varying purposes and lengths of time. It's not unusual to have several; there is so much more to learn. A mentor can make growth easier, because like so many of us, I tend to do better when I am accountable to someone else. Having Darcy in my life has been such a blessing! She holds my feet to the fire when they need it. I do it for her, too. I have now become skilled at doing it for myself.

Sometimes mentors appear in your life almost by magic; often they leave the same way. Nothing formalizing the relationship is ever needed.

I generally like to make things happen rather than wait for them to happen, so if I feel that I would like to be mentored, I ask. Try it. It is almost always a good experience. Find someone you admire who, in your judgment, can add something vital to your life, and ask him or her to mentor you. Be prepared to explain why you want a mentor in the first place and why you chose him or her. Outline what you have in mind, but work out the details together. Keep looking if you get a polite, "Sorry, I can't," and keep in mind that for most people, it's an honor to be asked.

When you find a good match, set up the mentoring arrangement as a trial, say for three months. Renew it if it is working well. Rethink the process and restart the search if not. Keep going until you find someone you click with, and continue until one of you wants to quit. If your organization is big enough but doesn't have a mentoring program in place, perhaps you could start one. It doesn't really matter where you find a mentor. All that matters is whether it works. Every study we have seen shows that it does, and all of our experience supports that. Start some serious buzz in your life. Get a mentor.

CLIENT FROM HEAVEN, CLIENT FROM HELL: COACHING YOURSELF

Self-coaching is not only possible, it happens all the time. We all do it, whether we're aware of it or not. Awareness, of course, is the key. If you choose to make your self-coaching a conscious process, you can achieve amazing things. I talk to myself. I tell myself what I need to hear, and what I may have forgotten. As with most complex endeavors, it's not always easy.

Sometimes I'm the client from heaven—cooperative, highly motivated, visionary, and action-packed. Sometimes I'm the client from hell— I ignore my own goals, lose sight of my vision, and am full of self-criticism or self-doubt.

Those negative behaviors are extremely rare these days, and almost nonexistent, because I have assimilated *The Ten Principles* so thoroughly that I can't help using them. They have become second nature. Controlling self-talk is where good self-coaching begins. Legitimate pride, enhanced self-esteem and amazing accomplishments is where it ends, if you do it right. However, it never really ends. Self-coaching is an ongoing form of entelechy—another way to control self-talk. It is a natural part of who we all are, urging us toward growth and fulfillment.

No one achieves anything worthwhile in this life on their own. As a species and as individuals, we need each other; need to help each other and try to improve things for the next generation—to leave a legacy that makes a positive difference. We accept help and we lend a hand to those coming after us. As I said at the beginning of this chapter, coaching and mentoring offer one of life's greatest and deepest pleasures. When done in a thoughtful and systematic way, it speeds up and sustains our growth.

USING *THE TEN PRINCIPLES* IN YOUR PROFESSIONAL LIFE
VITALITY STRATEGIES

THE ENERGY QUESTION

With the energy generated by enthusiasm, it feels as if you can do anything you put your mind to. No doubt you have experienced this yourself, many times. You tap into the power of your own vitality. You are more confident, get more done, connect and relate better to others, and think in more expansive, positive ways. But when you become ill or fatigued, things change. Positive energy is intermittent at best; at worst drained. Things that were important become peripheral, life fills up with too many things you have to do, and there isn't much you are excited about. A downward spiral starts. In light of this, it is important to learn how to safeguard your own energy supply.

The details of restoring or maintaining personal energy may differ from person to person, depending on temperament and preferences, but certain things are basic for almost all of us. Some of what follows will not be news to you, but when it comes to things that matter, reminders are always good. You need to do the things it takes to maximize your energy and vitality, and do them often enough to convert them into habits.

FIRST THINGS FIRST: REST, GOOD NUTRITION, AND EXERCISE

You would have to be living on another planet not to know that restful sleep, good nutrition and regular exercise are the cornerstones of health and vitality. It is certainly possible to exist on a steady diet of junk food, night after night of inferior rest, and a daily exercise plan that consists essentially of walking from your car to a building and back. Many people do just that. Those are the behaviors of benign neglect, and over time, they take a toll. They zap energy and erode health. We are a nation of overweight people suffering from a plethora of problems caused by our own bad habits.

You know what adequate rest means for you. Do what it takes to ensure it. You probably know what good nutrition is, too—eating a variety of fresh vegetables, fruits and whole grains every day, choosing lean meats or fish and poultry, limiting fats, sweets and empty calories, and aiming for few or no harmful additives or trans fats. What is stopping you from eating that way most of the time?

You know that you need to exercise regularly, too. Whatever your excuse for not exercising regularly has been, why not jettison it? If you start small but stay steady, it won't be long before it is so much a natural, normal part of your life that you'll be aware of your energy loss when you neglect it. Exercise energizes, and so does eating right and feeling rested.

Beyond this critically important Big Three, there are many other things you can do to keep your energy flowing. Here are several of my personal favorites. A few of Darcy's tried-and-true revitalizers are listed, as well:

- **Take solo time-outs.** Sabbaticals, retreats, R & R, no matter what you call them, they are important for maintaining energy, especially when you're around other people a great deal. This kind of time-out doesn't necessarily mean vacationing, unless you unplug, go alone, and have the right agenda. Stimulation is not the purpose; reflection is. Unless you spend time alone every now and then, it is easy to lose sight of yourself as an individual, apart from your roles and responsibilities. Next thing you know, you are feeling burned out, lost on a path you never intended or, far worse, trapped. A sabbatical is time to go one-on-one with yourself, ask important questions, see what answers come up, and decide what to do. Take one now and then. It is well worth it.

- **Indulge yourself.** If your nose is always to the grindstone and you're not having any fun, you're living too much in the future. Come up for air. Treat yourself to some time doing whatever you really love. Get a massage, go to a spa, share a good bottle of wine, see the show you've wanted to see, go rollerblading, get up a hike or a golf game with pals, or take your dream vacation. Don't do things that are supposed to be fun. Do things that really are.

- **Stay spiritually plugged in.** It doesn't matter what you believe in, but when belief falters, energy takes a fall. Everyone has doubts from time to time, and many people don't believe in God or divine provenance. However, nurturing a belief in something bigger than yourself makes life better and generates good energy for many people. If you have a spiritual connection, try not to neglect it. If you don't have one but think you might benefit if you did, do some investigation. Chances are excellent there is one out there that would work for you.

- **Give time to something you care about.** Give money, too, if you can, but if you want to feel some amazing Level Three energy blessing your life, get personally involved. Volunteer for something. I have always loved working with kids. What and who do you care about? Don't make giving time a one-shot thing, either; do it regularly. That way, you will really experience the amazing energy transfer that happens when you choose to serve something or someone beyond you and yours.

- **Diversify.** Sometimes we start to mistake the rim of our rut for the horizon. Don't let that happen to you. Every now and then, deliberately shake up your routines. Shower at night instead of in the morning. Get up an hour early. Take a different route to work. Hang out with people from other age groups, other religions, or other ethnic backgrounds. Get to know them better. See where you are alike and where you are different. Experiment with new foods, new sports, or new magazines. Eat as a family and one night a week or so, invite friends. Whenever you take yourself off autopilot, you generate fresh life energy. Try it and see.

- **Stop tolerating disorder.** I don't want to sound like your mother, but experience has taught me that it's true. If you have let your car, cubicle, office, house, yard, or anything else in your life become a chaotic mess—stop tolerating it. Throw out junk, give away things you don't use that are still useful, make files and piles, and find places for them. Think clean and uncluttered. It doesn't matter if it will become that way again in time. If it does, make it clear and clean again. Your life may be a mess, but your desk doesn't have to be. Start with a corner and keep going.

ENERGY, VITALITY AND PRODUCTIVITY

Your energy supply is an indicator of how strong, invigorated, or up to a task you feel. If you feel down, your enthusiasm diminishes and you tend to produce uneven or mediocre work. You miss things you might ordinarily see. Details slip through the cracks. Your ability to stick with a long or complex project may waver. When your energy is low, your productivity drops,

Tune in to your personal energy ebbs and flows, and try to plan your work around them. If you're a morning person, energized by the dawn of a new day and that first cup of coffee, do your most challenging work before noon. You will be better able to concentrate, make important decisions, and analyze what needs to be done. Or perform tasks that call for creativity or problem solving. When your energy is low, however, the work takes longer and feels harder. Results are more likely to be disappointing.

Some of us have higher natural energy levels than others. If yours feels lower than those around you, you can develop energy management strategies to make up the difference. Again, tune into your body and listen to what it tells you. As always, prevention is better than remedy, so try to keep from crashing in the first place. Make sure your body has a steady supply of blood sugar, but don't be deceived. Eating sugary snacks or empty calories won't give you what you need. If you eat refined carbohydrates when hungry—white flour, sugar, processed junk—you will get a brief surge of insulin, prompting an even bigger drop in blood sugar, which will leave you feeling edgy, irritable, and hungry. In turn, that will increase your appetite and drive you to eat the whole bag of cookies instead of just one. It's a vicious cycle that can really disrupt your entire day.

If you typically eat a muffin or donut in the morning or skip breakfast entirely, your blood sugar will spike, and then drop. A fast-food lunch compounds the problem. Soon you'll be hungry again, raiding the vending machines, and munching on whatever snacks you can lay your hand on. Instead, make a habit of eating a healthy breakfast that includes lean protein and whole grains. Grab a healthy snack every few hours throughout the day. Think protein and complex carbohydrates. Complex carbs—generally whole grains, beans, peas and root vegetables, are good carbs. They take longer to break down and deliver their nutrients to your body, and that slow burn provides a longer-lasting, steadier energy supply.

Use Energy Boosters

When you experience a low-energy period, make a conscious choice to change it. Instead of reaching for a caffeinated drink or candy bar, try one of these healthy energy boosters:

- **Protein smoothies.** If time doesn't allow you to eat well, try a protein shake. You can buy them ready made, or you can whip one up in the morning and take it with you in a Thermos. Protein powder from vegetable sources is readily available in health food stores or the natural foods section of better supermarkets.

- **Cold water.** This one sounds too easy, but it works. The face, neck and throat are sensitive areas. Splashing them with cold water acts as a stimulant, and temporarily diverts blood to your brain. Gargling with something ice cold can help, too.

- **Vitamin supplements.** While a well-balanced diet generally means you don't need them, not all diets are balanced, so vitamins can be useful. Vitamins C and E are good antioxidants, and a drink mix such as Emergen-C can provide an energy boost when you need one. Folic acid and B-complex can be helpful, too. Take a multivitamin every day, along with 1000-1500 mg of calcium, with vitamin D and magnesium added for ease of absorption.

- **Green tea.** Green tea is better than coffee for giving your energy a lift. It has enough caffeine to do the job, but not enough to make you shaky. As a bonus, it contains potent antioxidants and dilates bronchial passages, which improves oxygen flow.

- **Revitalizing oils.** Keep a bottle of peppermint oil in your desk or handbag. Inhaling this essential oil can clear your mind and raise your productivity. Other good oils include lemon, eucalyptus, juniper, orange and spearmint.

The difference between energy and lethargy can be as simple as noticing when your personal fuel gauge begins to point toward empty and taking prompt action. Take charge of your energy supply today. Learn to manage it wisely, and your "power outages" will be few and far between.

USING *THE TEN PRINCIPLES* IN
YOUR PROFESSIONAL LIFE
MANAGING CHANGE

NO SPEED LIMIT IN THE FAST LANE

Not long ago, only a few of us were living what we call "life in the fast lane." These days, whether we like it or not, the vast majority of us live and work there. Technological breakthroughs now happen in months and years instead of centuries. Calculations that once would have taken decades are now made in minutes. Communications that used to require months happen in seconds, and when it comes to rapid change, there's no end in sight. On the contrary, things will continue to speed up. The result of all this change is a future that is impossible to predict with any degree of accuracy, and for most of us, it's a life that is not only lived in the fast lane, it is in overdrive!

What does all this increasingly rapid change mean for you and your career or business? Perhaps your life has been moving so quickly that you haven't really had time to think about meaning. It is all you can do to simply keep up. If that is the case, you are not alone. Here is a snapshot of the big picture, which is, of course, still developing.

First of all, it's safe to say that most of us have adjusted fairly well to the relatively new development of computer-driven technology, which now plays a big part in our everyday lives. It's important to realize, however, that computer technology is still in its infancy. Speed and memory capacity are now doubling almost every eighteen months. What's more, a new breed of super intelligent computers is on the way—molecular computers that will make the PC on your desk seem primitive by comparison. These devices will be so small and incredibly smart that they will be the ones that design the computer generation that follows them, and those, in turn, will design the generation after that.

By the way, while we're talking about the big picture, keep in mind that the speeding up of change is not a recent development, although it may seem that way. In fact, it is a pattern that stretches back through history of the evolution of the earth. It is not easy to fully appreciate just how rapidly the entire process of evolution has been gaining speed. Let us give you an example that may help.

PUTTING CHANGE INTO PERSPECTIVE

Imagine a very tall building, about as high as New York's World Trade Centers used to be. Imagine that it has 108 floors. If street level represents the time when our planet was formed, which, most scientists agree, happened about 4.6 billion years ago, the first, single-celled organism didn't appear until the twenty-fifth floor. Multi-cellular organisms came on the scene at about the eightieth floor, and fish crawled out of the sea on the ninety-ninth. Dinosaurs roamed the earth on floors 104 to 107. Mammals finally put in their appearance on the very top floor. But the Neanderthals, with their bigger brains, simple tools and tribal culture didn't show up until the last quarter inch. The Renaissance happened in the top one-thousandth of an inch—less than the thickness of a coat of paint! The whole of what we call modern history occupies the thickness of a microscopic bacterium! Our era, the age of the microchip, rock 'n' roll, nuclear power, moon walks, global warming and the Internet is a layer almost too thin to measure.

With that picture in mind, you can begin to grasp the magnitude of what's happening to the rate of change on the planet, in this country, in your industry, whatever that is, and in your own life. But what does all this rapid change mean?

PREPARING TO ENTER NEW TERRITORY

I don't have the answer. No one does. All I can say with absolute certainty is that wherever we're going, we're going at an ever-increasing rate of speed. So it becomes important to ask ourselves how well are we equipped—as individuals and as organizations—to cope with this environment where change is happening constantly and the rate of change keeps speeding up? Are the skills we learned thirty, twenty, even ten years ago good enough to help us safely navigate this shifting sea of change? What should we be teaching our children about the best way to live in this high-velocity, computer-driven world? What should they be teaching us? How should we manage our resources so that we don't sacrifice the viability of our planet and the health of future generations for a quick profit today? How should we run our careers and businesses so that we not only survive, but thrive over time?

Ask 100 experts what's in store for us in the next decade or two, and they will come up with at least 100 answers. The wisest among them will admit they're just guesses, because every time something changes, many of the old questions start to become meaningless. Things are changing much too fast for anyone to predict the future. What's in store for you and for the leaders and managers of your organization? No one knows with certainty. We do know that in the next decades, we are going to be adjusting to the kind of rapid change that will make what's happened so far seem like slow motion.

Leaders in every field will be scrambling to keep up with new ways to reach and sell customers, new communication technologies, new markets and a barrage of new products and services. As a result, new kinds of training programs will need to be developed, because along with all the other changes, the rules of training will have changed, too. It used to be that a company could hire someone, train them once on how to do their job, and they were good to go. If a certain few employees had management potential, the company might provide additional training for them, but that was basically it.

Today, training has to be continuous. An entrepreneur or employee who isn't growing is falling behind, just as a company that isn't growing isn't simply standing still; it's losing ground. Whether you are a company, an employee or a free agent, if you are not operating on the leading edge, and if your employer, clients or customers don't perceive you that way, why will they keep doing business with you? If you are not leading edge, you are likely to find yourself teetering on the other edge, the one that leads to decline.

How Will Change Affect You?

Perhaps you already realize the importance of lifelong learning and continuous training. The idea I really want to convey is when it comes to change, and how it affects you—whether it's a source of stress or an opportunity for growth—depends on how you think and feel about it. People who resist change do so because they see it as a threat to their well-being, something rocking their boat. They are like that old horse you can lead to water. You can put them through the best training in the world, but you can't make these people see change as a good thing; something that is going to help the company grow and help them grow, if they are locked on to the idea that it is just another hassle they are forced to endure.

These are the people every employer would like to replace, if they could, with others who see change as an exciting opportunity—instead of something to guard against. Instead of replacing those folks, which can be costly and demoralizing, I challenge employers to *transform* them. More accurately, I challenge employers, employees and independent contractors everywhere to transform themselves!

The Ten Principles of Entelechy is a mind-opening, belief-changing experience that helps people think differently about change. It helps them recognize the beliefs that hold them back from taking advantage of change, and it gives them several practical, and immediately useful mental tools to help shift those beliefs.

Crisis = Danger + Opportunity

We are living in the most exciting, challenging and critical time in human history. This is true for the planet, for individual nations, for your industry as a whole, for your company, and it's true for you as an individual. As in any time of crisis, there is a great deal at stake. On the one hand, we have turmoil, but on the other hand, we have tremendous opportunity.

I challenge you to put *The Ten Principles* to work, day-after-day, week-after-week, year-after-year, in your office, your home and your heart. If you deliberately and systematically bring them into your life on a daily basis, they will keep working for you, no matter how quickly or radically things change.

In addition to bringing *The Ten Principles* to the workforce, here are ten things organizational leaders can do to ensure successful implementation of change efforts:

1. Involve as many stakeholders as possible in the change process.

2. Develop plans, but realize that they will likely need to be adapted and adjusted as needed

3. Educate managers. Make sure they know what to expect.

4. Make sure that every aspect of the organization is considered—employees, administrators, suppliers, strategic partners and, of course, customers.

5. Balance preparing for change and the need to move quickly. Getting people ready for change is important, but it should not take so much time and effort that they lose interest and motivation.

6. Provide plenty of training and staff development. These can include everything from *The Ten Principles of Entelechy* to focus groups to brown bag lunches where anticipated changes are discussed.

7. Recognize that change happens only through people. The emotional effects of change on employees need to be considered and understood by everyone affected. Understanding resistance and working with it is key.

8. Be prepared for "implementation dip." Things often get worse temporarily before improvement begins to appear.

9. Help all employees develop an intellectual understanding of the new practices. While anticipated outcomes are

important to convey, people also need to understand the underlying meanings and functions of the new practices.

10. Take the long view. Change takes time and should not be forced to occur too quickly.

USING *THE TEN PRINCIPLES* IN YOUR PROFESSIONAL LIFE
MANAGING YOURSELF

START BY SETTING GOALS

An executive I coached not long ago started his first session by saying he didn't want to talk about "that tired old goal-setting stuff." I asked whether he had any personal goals, apart from the goals of his organization. He said he did. I asked if they were written down. He said not really. Then I asked if he had a plan for how to achieve them. He said not really. Then I inquired as to how he was doing in terms of achieving them. He said he'd been too busy. Finally, I asked how he'd feel about getting those answers from a manager in his company. He shook his head, laughed, and we got started.

If you don't have clear, written goals or a plan for achieving them, it may be time to reconsider your rationale. People with written goals are more likely to achieve them than people who simply carry their goals in their minds. People who work systematically to achieve their goals are more likely to achieve them than people who just hope for the best.

No one would consider trying to manage a complex organization without a reasonable plan and a way to measure results. Almost everyone we encounter inside those organizations has no such plan in place for themselves. Like the exec mentioned above, they do have goals, but the goals tend to be either short-term or vague and there is generally no plan in place to achieve them. As a natural consequence, many of those goals end up buried under the mountain of day-to-day tasks and chores that take up our time, ignored or even forgotten.

BOOSTING GOAL ACHIEVEMENT

As I discussed in Part I, *The Ten Principles of Entelechy* teaches three techniques, that if used properly, can dramatically increase the likelihood of success in your change efforts. They are:

1. **Repeating and visualizing affirmations**

2. **Increasing positive self-talk**

3. **Decreasing or eliminating negative self-talk**

Hundreds of studies have proven that setting clear, specific, and challenging goals results in higher performance than not setting goals at all or setting goals that are vague and hard to measure. That's why, when you set a goal, it is important to make sure it has these two characteristics:

1. **It must be specific.** A specific goal should define a behavior and describe when and where it will occur. Instead of, "I will exercise as often as I can," a specific goal would be, "I exercise for thirty minutes or more, four times a week, either on the treadmill at the gym or by jogging in my neighborhood."

2. **It must be challenging, but attainable.** If your goal is too difficult, you will be more likely to give it up or procrastinate. If it is too easy, you won't feel much pleasure or see much progress when it is finally accomplished. Aim for something that feels like a stretch—neither easy nor impossible.

OVERCOMING OBSTACLES

When we try to change our behavior, we often find that our "default settings" tend to pull us back to our accustomed ways of doing things, even when the old ways weren't working well for us. If we can anticipate these potential obstacles to change, we can develop strategies to overcome them. In many studies of self-directed behavior change, people who had thought about possible obstacles and had a plan ready for how to deal with them, did much better than those who had no plan. So when you write your goals, list things that might prevent you from achieving them. After identifying these potential obstacles, think of several ways you could overcome each one.

TRACK PROGRESS, REINFORCE PROCESS, AND MANAGE RELAPSE

Keeping track of your progress is a key part of the process. Feedback is the breakfast of champions; it fuels motivation. Yours should involve two things:

1. Record goal-directed behavior as soon as possible afterward. Your count must be accurate and your system simple, and easy to use.

2. Identify what helps or hinders. At the end of each day, record what you did, how you might have done better, and what worked or didn't.

Like tracking, reinforcing keeps you motivated. It is a fundamental principle of behavioral psychology. Behaviors that are rewarded increase, while behaviors that are punished or ignored, decrease. So identify a few things that feel particularly gratifying for you to do or acquire and give them to yourself at intervals when you meet your goals, such as, at the end of your first successful day, week, month, quarter, and year. Withhold them if you miss a target.

Written contracts are also effective motivators. If you are serious about goal achievement, create an agreement spelling out what you will do, how you will track your efforts, how you will reward yourself for keeping the agreement, and when the agreement expires. Sign and date it. Read it weekly, as long as you need to.

The purpose of a self-management plan is to help you change certain behaviors in ways that last and become free-flowing parts of your life. Organizationally and individually, most change efforts begin with good intentions and initial success. Before long, though, we may find ourselves losing focus or returning to old ways. It takes time to build new habits. Relapse, especially at first, is fairly common. It may happen when we are under intense stress or operating on "autopilot." We simply revert to old programming and put ourselves back into an old comfort zone. The key to handling relapse is to Recognize and Remind. See it for what it is and remind yourself that there's a new program now.

Don't make the mistake of short-circuiting the change process due to a slip. If you have one, it doesn't mean change is impossible. Self-talk at every step of change, but especially after relapse, is critical. *Skip guilt trips, stay positive, and get strategic.* Good self-management means you know that learning about yourself and growing from what you learn are your most important tasks. Relapse offers a learning opportunity.

A relapse may mean that your self-monitoring system is too elaborate, your rewards too routine, or your goals too difficult. It can mean you are feeling emotionally drained or burned out, and in need of rest. Whatever it is, identify the causative situation or circumstance and develop remedies. If you could use some, ask for support; ask before the need becomes critical. And hang in there. You may manage many other enterprises or people in your lifetime, but none matters more than the job you do of managing yourself.

MAKE A LIST, AND CHECK IT MORE THAN TWICE

Here's a self-management checklist that can help guide you to better results. Every so often, review it to make sure you're doing what you need to do to ensure the best results.

1. **Set a specific goal.** Remember to specify exactly what you will do and when and where you will do it

2. **Track results.** Record your successes and failures, on a daily basis if that is appropriate. Write it all down.

3. **Share your intention and commitment.** Tell someone what your goal is. Check in with him/her at specific times to talk about how you're doing.

4. **Think small.** Trying to do too much too quickly is why many people fail at self-management. This is a big one; watch out for it.

5. **Beep at yourself.** If you find yourself getting distracted too often, use a device that beeps every so often to remind you of what you need to do.

6. **Impose a penalty for failure**. If you think it will help, keep it small, otherwise you may create tension, and you might even be tempted to quit.

7. **Get support.** It helps to put your self-management project on the agenda with someone you meet with regularly.

8. **Monitor your tracking**. Keep a record of your efforts, but consider asking your support person to monitor your recording, so it doesn't fall off.

9. **Eliminate distractions.** Watch out for that TV, phone, e-mail, or whatever else might get you off track. Your goal should come first.

10. **Persist.** Self-management may not work perfectly the first time you try it. Be prepared to "get back on the horse" as soon as possible if you fall off.

Remember, you do not demean yourself by employing a self-management system. If you persist in using these techniques, you will be in the company of some of the world's most productive people.

USING *THE TEN PRINCIPLES* IN YOUR PROFESSIONAL LIFE
VISIONARY LEADERSHIP

WHAT DOES IT MEAN TO LEAD?

In an information-driven, global economy of rapid change and ferocious competition, an organization needs not one but many leaders—leaders on every level throughout the system. The organization that has the greatest number of competent leaders is the one that enjoys the greatest competitive advantage.

What does it mean to be a competent leader these days? While today's leaders still need many of the traditional skills that marked leaders of yesterday, if they are going to succeed now and in the future, they need several new ones. Perhaps most important among them is a solid understanding of people.

Accordingly, we believe that the most important functions of a progressive business leader are these:

- To give the people inside the organization a clear, compelling vision of the organization's mission and purpose

- To help the people inside the organization see how what they do enables that vision and purpose

- To help the people inside the organization see how doing their best benefits not only the organization, but also them, personally.

Of course, there are other important things a leader must do, but these are paramount. If you do a good enough job with these three tasks, the people inside the organization will do the rest, and they will amaze you. They will take the vision and run with it.

A Vision is More Than Words

Many people believe that vision development is a straightforward task of articulating a vision statement and implementing it. Whether it is for a company or an individual, a team or a community, vision should not be a static thing, and developing it doesn't stop at one statement. To be truly useful and accurately reflect reality, vision must be more like an evolutionary process.

Leaders need to commit to continuous reflection and reevaluation, to doing more of what is sometimes called "purposeful tinkering." Through many small trials and errors, experiments and innovations, you keep coming closer to your vision, and tweaking the process as needed.

Whose Vision Is It?

Many people think an organization's vision should come from a strong leader with the imagination and charisma to drive change. I have worked with many leaders who shaped their organization's vision— some single-handedly. Coming from a respected, articulate leader, a distinctive personal vision can be more compelling than a something-for-everyone, group-produced stew. As long as people in the organization get excited about it, how the vision came about doesn't matter.

That said, there are good reasons to involve as many people as possible as soon as possible in the vision development process. After all, they are the ones who will have to translate abstractions into applications and bring the vision to life. They do this far better when they are actively involved in developing the vision from the get-go

Facilitate the Vision

No matter who creates it, organizational leaders must be the vision's chief instigators. Even the most empowered employees are not likely to spontaneously create a shared vision on their own. Leaders must also be the vision's principal promoters and guardians.

Often, leaders who have already adjusted to new ways of thinking underestimate the time it will take for others to adjust. The people in the trenches need an opportunity to examine their current thinking, develop a rationale for change, and entertain new ideas. *The Ten Principles of Entelechy* were created, in part, to provide that opportunity for our clients.

It is also crucial that the vision be operationalized. No matter how inspiring it sounds, vision withers unless it is expressed in action where the rubber meets the road—in policies, programs and procedures. Performance appraisals, hiring and staffing, bonuses and budgets must also be imprinted with the vision, or it will lose credibility. When you are a visionary leader, you must make sure that these things happen.

Above all, visionary leaders need to create a culture that welcomes change. The best leaders are steeped in it. They speak about the vision all the time, with conviction and enthusiasm. They encourage experiments, celebrate successes, and see failures as signs of life. They are determined in the face of inevitable problems and missteps, but not afraid to admit mistakes. Their clear sense of vision doesn't give them a magic bullet or make leadership a snap, but they are clear about its value. It makes dreams possible.

THE 80/20 RULE

Vilfredo Pareto, a nineteenth century economist, believed that most effects come from relatively few causes. He theorized that 80 percent of effects come from 20 percent of the possible causes. For example, 20 percent of the inventory items in the supply chain of an organization accounts for 80 percent of the inventory value.

Some leaders fall into the trap of focusing on the 80 percent of things that account for only 20 percent of the net worth. This is obviously a time-waster. Instead, a visionary leader should concentrate on the 20 percent that will have the greatest impact on the organization. It feels good to have small victories now and then from that easier 80 percent, but if most of their time and energy is spent on the few things that have the greatest impact, productivity will increase.

Inspire Your Organization. To *inspire* means "to breathe life into." Getting people to do something is much easier if they feel inspired. This is a visionary leader's job. These three actions will help leaders do that job well:

1. **Get excited.** In organizations where the leaders are enthusiastic about a project or change effort, the trickle-down theory is valid. If leaders are not communicating passion and excitement, how can they expect their people to feel that way?

2. **Involve employees in the decision-making process.** People who are involved in making decisions participate more enthusiastically than those who just carry out orders. Help everyone to contribute. Make sure they know that their ideas and opinions are valued. Listen to them and use their ideas when it makes sense. Reward participation and recognize it publicly.

3. **Understand the importance of people.** An organization may make a product or sell a service, but it is people who make it happen, and who ensure it happens well. A visionary leader's main responsibility is developing people and enabling them to reach their full potential. Although they come from diverse backgrounds, they all have goals they want to accomplish. Create a work environment where they can be all they want to be.

TRAIN AND COACH YOUR PEOPLE

Coaching and training are not the same things, even though the words are often used as if they were. Training provides information needed to do a job or learn new skills. Coaching helps people improve job performance, often by overcoming obstacles or solving problems. Coaching is more than telling people how to do something. It involves giving advice, skill-building, creating challenges, removing performance barriers, building better processes, and facilitating learning through discovery.

Although they are different, training and coaching go hand-in-hand. First you make sure that people are well trained so they develop a basic competency. Then you coach them by providing motivational pointers and tips for dealing with difficulties with the goal of helping them grow.

Both processes are more successful when leaders make sure that these things happen:

- Accurate assessment of current knowledge, skill and confidence levels.

- Definition of measurable objectives, often by breaking them down into step-by-step goals.

- Clear accountability. To promote this, involve the person or team in the decision making.

- Encouragement of peer coaching by reminding everyone that each has a stake in the other's success.

- Dealing with emotional obstacles by guiding people through change, pointing out ways that they may be holding themselves back, and offering support if they become confused or discouraged.

- Giving feedback by asking questions and pointing toward solutions rather than critiquing errors.

- Leading by example. Leaders and coaches must personally demonstrate the desired behaviors.

Using *The Ten Principles* in Your Professional Life
The Power of Diversity

Diversity is Our Destiny

When we think of diversity, we often think first of ethnicity and race, but diversity is much bigger and broader than that. It encompasses all of the human qualities that are different from our own or that occur outside the groups to which we belong. Diversity includes, but is not limited to, age, ethnicity, ancestry, gender, physical abilities/qualities, race, sexual orientation, educational background, geographic location, income, marital status, military experience, religious beliefs, parental status, and work experience.

It's important to realize that diversity is the natural order of things. Even though there is but one human species, the differences within it are staggering. Throughout the many centuries of human history, with the exception of identical twins, no two of us has ever looked alike, let alone thought or behaved alike. Even when we are raised in the same family, no two of us has the same experiences.

Diversity is neither small nor static. Diversity always makes things bigger and more interesting. It adds a mix of voices to the discussion, brings a number of points of view to the party, and puts more creative brain power to work on solving problems. A diverse group is the kind to have if you are trying to generate creativity, innovation and inspiration. It is the kind that really shines in times of crisis or rapid change, as well.

Diversity has become a hot issue because it has become a survival issue. If people of different races, religions, etc. can't learn to work together amiably and harmoniously, productivity suffers. If nations can't learn to work together amiably and harmoniously, or at least tolerantly, the entire planet suffers. Unless we change our ways, we will continue in an endless cycle of hatred and violence, adversarial to the bitter end.

To open ourselves to diversity, we must be able to hold a mirror up to ourselves and see what is really there. It is utterly familiar in one sense, yet may feel very scary in another.

RESPECTING DIVERSITY: NO STEREOTYPES APPLY

Respecting diversity doesn't mean treating everyone you meet in exactly the same ways. Stereotypes don't mean a thing these days, so cookie cutter approaches aren't useful. Instead, try to find and appreciate uniqueness in everyone. It helps to remember that we can all learn from each other.

Respecting diversity isn't about saying the "right" things or being unfailingly politically correct, either. It means focusing on listening, understanding, curiosity and empathy.

Diversity is not something we can always instantly embrace, either, especially if we were raised in a white-bread world or within an enclave of people who looked and behaved a lot like us. We can patiently and deliberately increase our awareness, maintain a flexible, open mind, and choose to be an adventurous, lifelong learner.

MANAGING DIVERSITY: THE PLATINUM RULE

To address diversity issues inside an organization, leaders must consider these two important questions:

1. Do the policies, practices, and ways of thinking within our organizational have a different impact on different groups?

2. What changes should be made to meet the needs of an increasingly diverse workforce and to maximize the potential of all our workers, so we can be well positioned for the demands of this century?

Most of us believe in the truth of the golden rule—Treat others as you want to be treated. Of course, this assumes that how you want to be treated is the same as how others want to be treated. If you look at this proverb through a diversity perspective, you will be led toward some intriguing and important questions. Is respectful treatment the same for everyone? Does showing respect mean greeting people with eye contact and inquiring about their health, or does it mean a brief nod and lowering your eyes? Does sharing personal information indicate friendliness, or does it mean a rude trespass of boundaries?

The answer, of course, is always the same…it depends. We may share similar values, such as respect or need for recognition, but how we show those values through behavior may be different. How do we know what different cultures prefer? Perhaps instead of using the golden rule, we could use the platinum rule: treat others as *they* want to be treated.

Many people think that fair treatment means that everyone is treated the same, but this may not work well with a highly diverse workforce. For example, employees with limited language or reading skills may be able to do their jobs well, but transmitting information in writing is probably not a good way to communicate with them. Someone like this who missed a memo containing essential information might feel that the process was unfair. A communication process that takes staff diversity into account might include extra time and effort to be sure that important information is understood. Such efforts on the part of supervisors and managers should be supported and rewarded as good diversity management.

Moving our frame of reference from an ethnocentric view (our way is the best way) to a culturally relative perspective (let's look at a variety of ways and see which is most useful in this situation) will help us to manage a diverse work environment more effectively.

How Well Do You Manage Diversity?

If you supervise others and can answer yes to more than half these questions, you are on the right track.

- Do you check out your assumptions before acting on them?

- Do you believe that there are a number of valid ways to accomplish a goal? Do you convey that to your people?

- Are you comfortable with everyone you supervise? Do you know what their goals are and how they like to be recognized?

- Can you give appropriate negative feedback to someone who is culturally or racially different from you?

- When you have job openings, do you use a diverse screening committee and make efforts to ensure you have reached a diverse pool of candidates?

- When orienting a new hire, do you not only explain job responsibilities clearly, but also orient the person to the organizational culture and unwritten rules?

- Do you make sure that existing policies, practices and procedures do not differentially impact different groups? If they do, do you change them?

- Are you willing to listen to constructive feedback from your staff about ways to improve the work environment? Do you implement staff suggestions and acknowledge contributions?

- Do you take corrective action when your people behave in ways that show disrespect for others, even if you are fairly sure no disrespect was intended?

- Do you make good faith efforts to meet any affirmative action goals?

- Do you have a good understanding of racism, ageism and sexism and how they may show up in the workplace?

- Do you make sure that assignments and opportunities for advancement are equally accessible to everyone who is qualified?

THE F WORD THAT CRIPPLES

If you don't yet understand the role fear plays in your life and how it stops you from opening up to others, now is a good time to learn. Most of us have been raised to trust the familiar and fear the strange or new. What's more, we have learned to judge the familiar as superior. Our brains have become expert at categorizing, labeling and generalizing data so we can deal quickly with the natural diversity of life. As a result, we stereotype without meaning to. It's a knee-jerk reaction and, unfortunately, we all do it.

Fear of differences and the biases and prejudices that accompany it are habits of thought. They are reinforced by filtered perceptions, incomplete education, personal experiences, hearsay, "tribal" knowledge, our culture, and of course, the media. These habits are formidable obstacles; but no fear or bias can compete with a truly open, curious mind.

CULTIVATE CURIOSITY

Curiosity invites change. When we are curious, we see new possibilities. Maybe they have always been there, but we built scotomas to them. However, once we open our minds to those possibilities, we just keep discovering more. Our reticular activating systems start shifting information from our unconscious to our conscious minds. We start to notice, often for the first time, everyone's unique contributions, personalities, knowledge, strengths and weaknesses. In other words, we let them in.

A single storyline about anyone can't possibly capture the complexity and richness of their life. When we break through the boundaries of our own old habits, attitudes, beliefs, perceptions and expectations, we invite diversity and all the advantages it brings. It is more like a garden salad than a melting pot, with many tastes and textures. Each is unique, distinct, and with the right dressing, complimentary.

DIPLOMATS OF DIVERSITY

A curious mind cannot rely on stereotypes. They blur, distort and demean. Cultural heritage aside, we are all individuals and should be treated as such.

How might your opinions and biases change if you:

- Learned a new language?

- Traveled to a country you are unfamiliar with?

- Joined an organization that includes people who stretch your comfort zones?

- Encouraged cross-functional teams inside your organization?

- Saw everyone you met as a teacher who could expand your awareness?

- Invited foreign-born neighbors or acquaintances to dinner?

- Tried to make friends from different backgrounds?

Be curious. Venture into new territories. Value human differences. Celebrate humanity. Respect others. Focus on the horizon, not the old familiar, and enjoy the journey—discovery, new experiences, and personal growth. Embrace diversity by networking across cultural biases and getting people from diverse backgrounds and ethnic heritages to work together for common goals. Challenge biased statements when you hear them, and help others become more culturally sensitive and savvy. In a world where cultural differences have ignited and fed devastating conflicts, we must *all* become diplomats of diversity.

Using *The Ten Principles* in Your Professional Life
The Ten Principles at Work

Adjust Your Focus

Whether your professional life currently feels like a challenge or a walk in the park, two things are certain: 1) You are going to go through a lot of changes in the months and years ahead, and 2) More than anything else, the thing that will determine how it all comes out is where you choose to focus your energy and attention.

If you've ever gone through a time of great turmoil or trouble in the past and found yourself pushed to your limit, you may have discovered that your limit was actually farther out than you thought. Looking back, perhaps you can identify a defining moment or turning point when you became very clear about what you wanted and did not want. Never again, you may have said, will I get myself into a situation like this. Never again will I have to worry like this about money. Never again will I risk my physical or emotional health. Never again will I put my family last and my job first. Never again will I take my safety and security for granted. Most of us have been there. I know I have.

At these moments, your focus shifted, clarified and narrowed. You used that clear focus as a catalyst to propel yourself into a new and different way of being. That kind of refocusing can lead to tremendous, lasting positive change in your career, because there is nothing, absolutely nothing, more powerful than a clearly focused, and determined mind. What needs to follow such determination, of course, is willingness to do the work.

CHANGE TAKES WORK

It isn't always easy to stay the course when it comes to building a successful, and satisfying career. It certainly isn't just a matter of repeating affirmations, developing a more positive attitude, and—presto!—your life becomes an incredible success story, filled with plenty of money, oceans of promotions, and just about everything you ever wanted.

We at Entelechy teach the techniques of affirmation, visualization and positive thinking in *The Ten Principles* curriculum because they are powerful tools, and we believe everyone can benefit from knowing how to use them, personally and professionally. But, make no mistake, they aren't magic wands. To get where you want to go over the long haul, to stay the course when times get tough, to pick yourself up and start over when you have had the rug pulled out from under you—requires you to expend the effort.

Creating the life and the career you want will require determination and persistence, day after day, month after month, year after year. It won't always be smooth sailing, although it is true that as you grow in experience and hone your skills, the process does get easier. Yes, it's filled with satisfaction, joy, and the thrill of achieving a difficult goal, and then going on to set and achieve many others. Yes, it offers lasting, high-level happiness in the long run. However, it also has its share of disappointments, heartaches and frustration.

WHEN THINGS FALL APART

Every once in a while, you will really be put to the test. Maybe you'll lose your job. Maybe you'll even get fired. Maybe your industry will be besieged by scandal or largely replaced by computers. There will be days when you will doubt your ability to hang in there—days when all you want to do is quit. You will have days when you are sure that your get-up-and-go has gone for good. But you absolutely can do it. You can create a successful professional life, no matter what happens to you, no matter what happens to the economy, and no matter what happens to your company. You can do this...if you:

- Stay focused on your long-term vision

- Are flexible, open to change and to learning new skills

228

- Control your self-talk

- Seek help when you need it

- Plan for it, visualize and affirm it, and work for it

- Exercise the self-discipline needed for the long haul, and

- Refuse to quit.

Keep in mind that it won't always be something extremely difficult that presents the biggest challenge. Your biggest challenges may often come from the routine, day-after-day grunt work that you really don't enjoy and may have a tendency to postpone or skip. If you patiently persist in doing what you need to do, your efforts will eventually pay off and you will end up with something great to smile about.

INCREMENTAL CHANGE MOVES MOUNTAINS

In the same way, the changes that you make in your life—all those positive, focused things that you do on a daily basis—may seem small, and even insignificant for a while. As the old saying bids us to remember, "A journey of ten thousand miles starts with a single step." Similarly, most major changes happen in small increments. When done consistently, small things add up.

The value of an experience, *any* experience, is up to you. When something bad, even something really terrible happens to thwart your career plans, you can react as you may have been conditioned to react—with defeat, frustration, helplessness, hopelessness, and anger. Or you can decide that you will salvage something from the loss.

If you're having an experience that you are not enjoying, change it, if you can. If you can't change the factors involved, you can certainly change your response. Decide to accept it for what it is. Learn from it and grow. What you allow yourself to think about during any experience determines the effect that it has on you. Bad times can't last when you banish negative, self-doubting, hopeless or discouraged thoughts.

The Illusion of Certainty

Being too sure of anything is usually a mistake. Change is the first rule of life. As a consequence, certainty is generally an illusion. Even your beliefs and core values are likely to change over time. Believe it or not, even your memories of the past may change, as well. Being too sure of anything can stop you from growing. Are you sure you have found your life's work? Maybe not. Are you positive you will never go back to school? Never say never. Are you certain of where you are going in your organization? You could be wrong. Do you know how much success you are capable of creating? Don't be so sure.

We all like to be certain of who we are and what we know. It helps us to feel confident and comfortable. Locking onto any idea of "what is" can be dangerous because it means we are locking out a world of other possibilities at the same time. How might it benefit you to keep an open mind about some of the things you're sure of, or some of the ideas that may be limiting you or holding you back? If you remain open to new possibilities, that state of receptiveness alone can change things for you.

If you make them an integral part of your life, *The Ten Principles of Entelechy* can be used to address any issue, solve any problem, and get you anywhere you want to go. If you develop the attitude of gratitude and focus on the things you want to achieve, the things you want to improve, the things you can give and the things you love, you will not only stay the course, you will cross the finish line with the professional life you have always wanted.

Using *The Ten Principles* in
Your Professional Life
Ethics Nine to Five

What is Ethical?

Ethics are principles of behavior. They tell us how to act in ways that will meet the standards set by our values. When our behavior is consistent with our values, and our values conform to commonly accepted moral principles, we are behaving ethically. When our actions are not congruent with our values or are considered immoral by society, we are acting unethically.

Defining what is ethical is not up to an individual, a particular group or a particular organization. If it were, one could argue that what Saddam Hussein did while he ruled Iraq was ethical, since his actions conformed to his own definition of right and good. While the ethics of our decisions and actions must be defined by society, individuals and organizations may still create and follow codes of behavior that express society's ethics in their own words and ways.

Workplace Ethics: Threat and Opportunity

The post-Enron/WorldCom environment of public distrust and tightening regulation exposes corporations to both new threats and new opportunities. The principal threat is obvious—disastrous loss of shareholder value as a consequence of real or perceived unethical practices or behaviors. The opportunity may be less apparent, but is equally real—to reform corporate practice and norms to gain strategic advantage and minimize risk.

Rethinking and restating corporate purpose in terms of social needs is an effective way to distinguish your company from the competition, promote public trust and ultimately increase stakeholder (not just shareowner) value. The goal must be not only to do well, but also to do good. In that respect, it is important to balance the interests of all stakeholders by practicing enlightened self-interest—economically, competitively and socially.

CORPORATE ETHICS: A MATTER OF TRUST

No matter what you manufacture, sell or service, your company is in the trust business. If you sell cars, motorcycles, airline tickets, food, pharmaceuticals, children's toys, cosmetics, or countless other products, you know that if people don't trust their safety, they won't buy your products or services. If you are a bank, brokerage, insurance company or accounting firm, you know that if you aren't trusted, your profits will dry up. If you accept credit cards as payment, your customers must trust you with their account numbers. Whoever you are and whatever you do, without trust you are out of business.

Once consumer trust is damaged, it takes enormous effort to regain it. Sometimes, despite Herculean attempts, it simply can't be done. It is not simply an exercise in damage control, as Enron and Arthur Andersen came to realize. Together, these two companies became symbols for a series of incidents that make a compelling case for the importance of trust. Ethical behavior engenders and deepens trust.

THE HIGH COST OF LOW ETHICAL STANDARDS

When leadership practices are not aligned with the organization's ethical standards, it can result in:

- Employees ignoring ethical standards to pursue results at any cost

- Loss of organizational credibility as people see standards being disregarded

- Decreased productivity as employees feel less committed and comfortable

- Employees not believing they can legitimately raise ethical questions at work

- Ethics guidelines seen as window dressing, and not legitimate operating principles

- Increased conflict as people are expected to violate their personal standards

- Increased stress as the work environment becomes ethically incongruent

- Loss of overall effectiveness, and inevitably, profits, as ethical conflict undermines other aspects of the operation

ETHICAL LEADERSHIP: ROOTS AND RESULTS

Ethical leadership begins with a willingness to face reality, search for the truth and courageously tell it to others, but it doesn't end there. Ethical leaders are also responsible for finding hope in dark times and inspiring action that increases not only the benefits to themselves and those they lead, but also to something bigger—the common good. This doesn't always make them popular, but ethical leadership is not about popularity. It's about integrity and service for the greater good.

Here are six things organizational leaders can and should do to ensure that their businesses grow in ways that are both profitable and ethical:

1. **Develop** consensus on a revised statement of corporate mission/purpose that includes your company's ethical foundation and intentions.

2. **Clarify** the role of profit in your business equation. David Packard, co-founder of Hewlett-Packard, once commented, "Profit is not the proper end and aim of management—it is what makes all of the proper ends and aims possible."

3. **Communicate** the distinction between old and new purpose, values, and behavior to all stakeholders—

233

employees, customers, vendors, and the general public. Every leader should know what the organization's ethical standards are and how they are expected to support them.

4. **Set** a strong and unmistakable personal example. Get clear about what ethical behavior is, and then walk the talk, every step of the way.

5. **Provide** systems to support the ethics-related actions of leaders, including policies that recognize the value of ethical leadership practices and structures that allow employees to raise ethics concerns without fear of disapproval or reprisal.

6. **Revise** your organization's management measurement and reward system so that when the values and ethics your organization preaches are practiced by managers, they are appropriately acknowledged and rewarded.

NUDGING THE WORLD

Playwright Tom Stoppard says, "Words are sacred… If you get the right ones in the right order, you can nudge the world a little…" Accordingly, the way organizational leaders choose to communicate their philosophy of corporate responsibility is important. Fortunately, it is easy to connect bottom-line business priorities with corporate responsibility practices and terminology, if you give it a bit of thought.

Cost control and risk management strategies can dovetail nicely with proactive environment, energy and safety policies. Attracting and retaining human capital in an increasingly knowledge-based economy goes hand-in-hand with employee diversity and ongoing training. Market development plans can take growing social causes into account. The value of your reputation and brand meshes with the value of soft assets on your balance sheet.

Perhaps most important is a deep-rooted shift in priorities. Just as individuals must learn to value long-term well-being over the lure of today's tempting indulgences, long-term organizational health and vitality must become more important than short-term profits. Until this mindset is firmly entrenched throughout the organization, serious breaches of ethical boundaries can be expected. Once the long view becomes as important as quarterly returns, organizations can do great things. They can ensure their own competitiveness and well-being at the same time they nudge the world toward becoming a better place.

Using *The Ten Principles* in
Your Professional Life
Winning Teams

When is a Group a Team?

A team is any group of people with a high degree of interdependence, all working toward achieving the same goal or completing the same task. They may have different functions within the team, but their goal is a common one that can't be achieved independently. Of course, many groups have common goals, but the key is interdependence. The members of a team agree on a goal and recognize that to achieve it, they must work together. The more effectively they work together, the more likely it is that they will accomplish what they have set out to do. Sports teams are, obviously, a perfect example.

Types of Teams

These days, the three most common kinds of teams in business are functional teams, self-directed teams, and cross-functional teams.

Functional teams are most common. They are composed of a leader and his/her direct reports, and they operate on a military model, more or less. Issues of authority, responsibility, working relationships and decision-making paths are clearly defined. Functional teams work best in stable industries with predictable markets.

Self-directed teams are somewhat more difficult to define. Most often, a self-directed team is a group of people who share responsibility for a well-defined unit of production, such as an airplane fuselage, or a service, such as a fully processed loan application. They have the authority to plan, develop, implement, control and improve any or all processes.

Self-directed teams are also found in traditional organizations, but they are especially well suited to startups or companies with a base of participative management and a history of employee involvement.

Cross-functional teams are part of the quiet revolution that is sweeping across organizations today, and they can be found in a wide variety of industries. Generally, a cross-functional team has a clearly-defined purpose. It is composed of people who represent a variety of functions within the organization and whose combined efforts are needed to achieve that purpose.

Cross-functional teams are most often used to solve a problem that impacts multiple parts of the organization, to improve a work process that crosses organizational lines, to coordinate ongoing processes or activities that cross organizational boundaries, or to accomplish tasks that require a breadth/depth of knowledge, skills and experience. Cross-functional teams are most effective in companies with fast-changing markets or those that value adaptability, speed, and focus on responding to customers' needs.

CROSS-FUNCTIONAL TEAM CULTURE

Constructing a cross-functional team is not an unduly complex process. Defined below are the customary objectives.

1. Select team members with an optimal mix of skills and expertise.

2. Clarify team objectives and outcomes.

3. Identify the roles and responsibilities of each team member.

4. Use the knowledge of the entire team to determine strategies and solutions to accomplish objectives.

5. Determine timelines and action steps.

6. Provide team members with training in teamwork skills, such as communicating, listening, and facilitating.

7. Periodically evaluate the team's functioning.

Building an effective cross-functional team is not quite so simple. Significant differences between team members can stand in the way of getting the job done. Consequently, it is important that everyone sees the team as more than just a joining of functions. They must also realize that it is a complex blending of real people with different histories, styles, skills and priorities.

The quality of the team's results depends on many things, but paramount among them is their ability to communicate effectively and integrate individual resources, knowledge and perspectives. This requires a shift in point of view—from "my" function, goals, values and beliefs to "our" function, goals, values and beliefs. Success must mean team success. Rewards must mean team rewards. If the team should fail, the failure is shared by all, equally.

Most teams, particularly cross-functional teams, are made up of people from many walks of life, ethnicities and cultures. They have different emotional maturity levels, educational backgrounds, skill sets, expectations, belief systems and previous team experience. This kind of diversity can be extremely useful. It can also make effective communication challenging. Team members often assume that communication has taken place when it hasn't. Poor communication can cause strained relationships, lack of focus, undetermined agendas and misused time.

FACILITATING EFFECTIVE TEAM COMMUNICATION
Excellent team communication is the product of training, practice and hard work. Leaders need to create a climate within which team members can communicate openly, promptly, accurately and regularly. Effective communication allows a team to stay fine-tuned for exceptional performance.

Here are five things a team leader—or team members themselves—can do to facilitate the kind of communication that keeps a team on track.

1. **Build strong team relationships.** Solid team relationships can exist without members becoming best buddies. Their bond is primarily their dedication to a

239

clear, common, and compelling purpose. When team members do not experience solid relationships, their trust level rapidly declines. Trust and communication spiral downward (or upward) together.

2. **Model active listening.** Many team leaders want to be heard, but they don't listen well. Team members will connect with team communications to the same degree that team leaders value the team's input.

3. **Put new ideas on trial.** Team members must challenge each other to investigate the potential up and down sides of new ideas. Winning teams take time to ensure that their ideas truly serve the team's purpose and fall within the organization's mission.

4. **Educate everyone.** Never assume that because a team is made up of intelligent, highly motivated people, that they know how to communicate effectively. Training must be provided, and opportunities for practice and review should be plentiful and ongoing.

5. **Engage everyone.** Team leaders and members must remember to reach out to the edge of the group, where the quieter, more reflective members tend to be found, and proactively seek input from those who may not feel that "this is their area." This takes advantage of the benefits of diversity, and conveys that all members' input are valued, and builds trust.

TEAMS MUST LEARN TO TRUST

A critical dynamic of teams, particularly cross-functional teams, has to do with trust. If a team project is assigned to a single discipline group (marketing, engineering, etc.), each team member is likely to have the ability to check the work of other team members.

In collaborative cross-functional projects, on the other hand, each member brings to the table knowledge and processes that cannot be checked in detail by other members. The marketer can't really check the engineering calculations, and the engineer is rarely equipped to check the allocation decisions of the accountant. This reality may affect team performance. Trusting each other becomes a critical team dynamic—one that requires time, effort and, very often, training.

USING *THE TEN PRINCIPLES* IN YOUR PROFESSIONAL LIFE
WHAT HAPPY COMPANIES KNOW

When I discovered the book, *What Happy Companies Know*, I couldn't wait to spread the word. Drawing on the new positive psychology, it outlined the research that had been done and applied it to building organizations, particularly businesses. It painted a compelling picture of how certain practices—practices that engendered a satisfied, and fulfilled workforce—were the same ones that helped companies compete successfully and thrive. I sincerely hope its publication marks the beginning of a trend. If so, it's time. I have been teaching it for years.

WHY PEOPLE QUIT

Today, there is no such thing as job security and new faces in the organization are the rule, not an exception. Those who stay with a company more than a year or two are not always the people doing the best job; they are often the ones who have little or nothing to offer another employer.

Customers who keep buying, however, are uncomfortable with high turnover. They don't like losing familiar contacts or doing business with a company whose face keeps changing. When employees they know and trust leave, clients and customers often elect to go with them.

No two companies are exactly alike. The best way to find out why employees are leaving is to survey their opinions and intentions; the overwhelming majority tell the truth and are grateful to be asked. It can also be enlightening to take a look at global survey databases. It turns out that there is a clear relationship between job satisfaction (i.e., belief that one's skills and abilities are being used, that the company has a clear sense of direction, and that its managers are competent) and intention to leave.

What's more, pay, often considered the single most important factor by employers, doesn't rank high on the list of employees' concerns. Even though they may talk about money and want to be paid what they believe they are worth, when it comes to staying with a company and doing their best, money is not an important motivator for most employees.

NINE REASONS WHY EMPLOYEES STAY

People want to find meaning and satisfaction in their work. They get those important things from noneconomic factors, such as using their skills in a challenging effort, feeling valued and being led by capable managers who have a clear sense of direction.

Organizational leaders need to know how their people feel. They need to know who is dissatisfied and why. Often the best way to find out is to conduct a confidential survey and act promptly on the results, before employees decide to take action themselves by going someplace else.

In the meantime, here are nine reasons why we believe the best people remain the best people in organizations of every kind:

1. **They know their managers care.** Bosses who take a genuine interest in helping employees further their careers and do well on the job make a big difference in job satisfaction ratings. When managers care, it shows.

2. **They believe they can grow.** People who can't satisfy their need for career growth inside the company eventually resign. New assignments, even if temporary, are a great way to help people stretch. Likewise is training that challenges them to think differently.

3. **They see where the company is going, and they want to go.** Having a clear vision is a good start. Making

sure managers understand and promote it is important, too, but every employee should know it like the back of their hands, and leaders must walk their talk.

4. **They know you value and measure soft skills.** Don't just pay lip service to the idea of genuinely caring about your people. Tie career coaching to manager compensation, and document it when it happens.

5. **They think their managers are great.** Conduct 360-degree performance appraisals. Mediocre managers must know how and why they need to improve. If they don't improve, replace them with people who can get the job done—people who help those they manage to grow and develop.

6. **Poor performance isn't tolerated.** When they see that poor performance is tolerated, good people become resentful or frustrated and end up walking out. Underperforming employees should be coached and given a fair chance to improve. If improvement doesn't happen, they should be given notice.

7. **They benefit from training.** To keep good employees happy, provide training that adds to their job satisfaction or skill base. Find out what people really want and give it to them. If possible, training should happen on company time and be evaluated afterward by the participants. If a training course gets rave reviews, repeat it for others. If it tanks, yank it.

8. **Personal and team recognition is the norm.** Don't make the mistake of thinking that people who are well paid don't need strokes. Make sure that individuals and teams who go the extra mile get noticed and applauded. Make knowing what "the extra mile" means and make spotlighting it a part of every manager's job.

9. **They feel like insiders.** People want to be in the loop. In many happy companies, top executives make

themselves available for discussion and dialogue. In-house newsletters, company-wide gatherings, social events and training in skills that can be used both on and off the job help keep work and personal life connected.

WHAT MAKES THEM SO HAPPY?

Happy companies see reality clearly, including the not-so-pleasant parts, but they choose to address it positively. They perceive opportunities as well as obstacles, and they lead with values, optimism and fairness. They promote creativity and pragmatism. They avoid the reactive, unthinking decisions that people make when they are driven by anxiety and fear.

Several of the specific characteristics of happy companies have already been covered in previous chapters, including the importance of a shared, value-driven vision and a mission that provides meaning and purpose to those who work toward it. A few others deserve special mention:

- **Their self-talk is positive.** How people talk matters hugely inside an individual's mind and inside an organization. In happy companies, the self-talk is constructive, inspiring and hopeful.

- **The climate is one of appreciation and good humor.** People focus on what's working and what's going well as they work toward a better tomorrow. They laugh and have a playful spirit. At the same time, they get an amazing amount of work done.

- **They support each other.** People inside happy companies help each other out, on and off the job. They show kindness and consideration to each other as a matter of course—behavior that is modeled from the top down.

- **They routinely go above and beyond.** "That's not my job" is something you are not likely to hear inside a happy company. Instead, people do whatever it takes to get the job done, as long as "whatever" is ethical.

- **The focus is on opportunities.** This means they are forward-thinking, and forward-looking people. They explore, experiment, and take risks. Mistakes are examined to learn from, and successes are examined to replicate and teach.

- **They play fair.** Integrity is expected. Honesty and fair treatment are the norm. Ethics are discussed, codified and brought to life in every transaction. For these reasons, people are able to trust each other.

- **Continuous improvement and lifelong learning are encouraged and rewarded.** Meaningful training and mentoring programs are common, and employee development is central to the organizational culture.

Using *The Ten Principles* to Enrich Your Professional Life

Professional Affirmations

The following affirmations have been created to support the material in Part III. Use them as guides for writing your own or borrow them as is. Remember to visualize and *feel* what you describe; believe in the truth of the words, and repeat the process often.

- Having a clear vision for my future energizes and excites me.

- It feels great to know where I am going and why I want to go there.

- Because my values are clear, I spend my time wisely.

- My personal life and my professional life complement each other perfectly.

- I take good care of myself, so I have an abundant energy supply.

- I am a lifelong learner who truly enjoys helping others.

- I love what I do, so I keep getting better at it.

- My self-talk at work is positive, optimistic and helpful.

- Change offers me new opportunities to learn and grow, so I embrace it.

- My self-management system works beautifully because I use it.

- I bring *The Ten Principles* to work with me because they help me succeed.

- I bring a sense of humor and genuine enjoyment to my work.

- I am curious and respectful about people from different backgrounds.

- I can be a strong leader or a smart follower, as the situation requires.

- Ethical behavior is a central part of who I am.

- I truly enjoy striving for excellence in my work and work relationships.

- I care about helping everyone around me to succeed.

PART IV
THE SPIRIT OF ENTELECHY

The Spirit of Entelechy
The Keys to Happiness

What's Your HQ?

How happy are you these days? How happy have you been in the past? How high would you say your overall HQ (Happiness Quotient) is?

According to polls, Americans aren't happier now than they were fifty years ago, even though prosperity has increased and crime decreased, the air is cleaner, living quarters are larger and the overall quality of life is better. So what does it mean to be happy? What kinds of people are happy? What is it that makes them happy?

Researchers say that happiness is about 50 percent genetic, although that theory may be changing. What we do with the other 50 percent depends on a combination of the environment and what psychologists call human agency, which simply means our ability to choose or decide. This book and all of Entelechy's work, including *The Ten Principles,* centers around that other half—the part you can control. But *do* you control it?

The Bad News, and the Good News

If your HQ is on the low side, take heart. Psychologists have recently handed the keys to happiness to us, but many people either haven't heard the news or stick to their melancholy ways because of mistaken beliefs. They are convinced that good looks and money buy happiness, and no wonder. That is what they have been conditioned to believe by a media-fueled, consumer-driven culture, and very often, by parents who believed the same thing. It turns out that beautiful people are no happier than the rest of us, and money only increases happiness if it is used to lift people out of poverty. After that, bigger paychecks don't correlate with an improved sense of well-being.

A more reliable route to happiness is called "flow," an engrossing state that is stimulated by creative or playful activity, according to psychologist and author, Mihaly Csikszentmihalyi. Athletes, musicians, writers, gamers and religious adherents know the feeling well. It comes less from what you do than from how you do it.

Another path to a higher HQ is via a road you never walk alone. Many studies have shown that the happiest people are likely to be those with strong interpersonal connections, including valued friendships. Altruism and gratitude help you be happier, too. "There are selfish reasons to behave in altruistic ways," says Gregg Easterbrook, author of *The Progress Paradox: How Life Gets Better While People Feel Worse* (Random House, 2004). "Research shows that people who are grateful, optimistic and forgiving have better experiences with their lives, more happiness, fewer strokes, and higher incomes. If it makes the world a better place at the same time, this is a real bonus."

THREE THINGS THAT WORK

The University of Pennsylvania's Martin Seligman, whose research on learned optimism and positive psychology has been widely accepted and quoted, has a great deal to say about happiness these days. According to Seligman, there is good scientific evidence that three activities can make us lastingly happier and reduce depressive symptoms. He has dubbed them, "The Gratitude Visit, Three Good Things and Using Your Strengths."

- **The Gratitude Visit.** Think of a person in your life who has been kind or helpful to you but whom you have never properly thanked. Write a detailed letter to that person, explaining in concrete terms why you are grateful. Then, visit him or her—in person, if possible—and read your letter aloud.

  A gratitude visit can generate its own momentum and create a wonderful chain of events. The people you visit and thank begin thinking about who deserves thanking in their own lives, and they make their own pilgrimages. It happens to the people they visit, too. Perhaps such visits will create an ever-greater ripple of gratitude and joy that keeps on going for generations. A woman in one of our seminars told the group that she wrote her gratitude letter to someone who had died, so she took it to the cemetery and read it aloud. "I cried tears I didn't know I had," she said, adding that she felt forever changed by the experience.

- **Three Good Things.** Every night for one week, describe in writing three good things, large or small, that happened during the day. Next to each thing on your list, answer the question, "Why did this good thing happen?" Try to answer thoughtfully. Don't say, "I guess it was just one of those things," or "Who knows?" or even "Probably a happy accident." Look deeper. Search for internal causes as well as external. You don't need to be certain that what you write is true, but try to be insightful, objective and logical.

- **Using Your Strengths.** By whatever method you wish (try the "Signature Strengths" survey at www. authentichappiness.com) to assess yourself and decide on your top five strengths. Then, use these five strengths in new ways every day for one week. Opportunities to do this may arise spontaneously, but it is best to plan ahead. Try to decide beforehand what you are going to do. Record what you did and how it went.

If you are willing to take on the challenge of these activities, you are likely to raise your happiness quotient. Why not try one? In fact, if you really want to boost your HQ, try all three.

POSITIVELY POWERFUL

We are all familiar with the different intensity levels that negative emotions have. We know the difference between annoyance, anger, rage and hatred. We know the difference between feeling concerned, worried, afraid and terrified. Most of us also know that the more intense and powerful our negative emotions, the more suffering they cause for ourselves and others. Strong negative feelings such as hatred, terror and greed lead to terrible results in the external world. However, positive emotions are every bit as powerful.

Positive emotions have gradations or levels, too, though not many people seem to realize it. There is a wide range of happiness—from brief, mild pleasure through intense passion to deep contentment. There is also a range of compassion—from mild concern to strong feelings of connection and caring. Unfortunately, many people associate love and compassion with weakness. They believe that if they wish to be perceived as strong, they must also be feared. Consequently, they often express contempt and anger, but suppress any impulses toward kindness or more tender feelings. Eventually, there is nothing left to suppress.

Once you understand and have personally experienced the great value and healing power of love and compassion, you are almost always motivated to increase them. The earlier in life it happens, the better. The great spiritual traditions of the world have always taught it; now a large body of scientific research backs it up. These feelings heal and create lasting happiness. When you deliberately develop your love and compassion for others, you also benefit.

Lazy = Unhappy?
What stops people from being happy? What's the biggest obstacle? There are many answers, such as, low self-esteem, limiting beliefs, negative self-talk, poor self-image, a desire to punish themselves for some reason, and so on. All of these are valid and worth considering, but another answer stands out, perhaps because it is so simple.

A few years ago, I was sitting on a kitchen stool holding a glass of wine one evening. I was talking with my mother, who was whipping up a batch of ravioli. I asked her what she thought it was that held people back from being truly happy. Mom, who was and still is one of the hardest working people around, looked at me, shook her head, and made a sound, "Hrmph!" Then she said, "Lazy," and went back to kneading her dough.

I let it go at the time, assuming she had someone specific in mind, possibly me! Later, thinking it over, it occurred to me that she was probably right. It may well be nothing more complicated than laziness that holds many people back from doing the things that lead to happiness.

If unhappiness is our default condition, is it because it takes less effort? It is always easy to find things to complain about, and things that aren't the way we'd like them to be. To be miserable, we don't even need to get off the couch. On the other hand, unless you're one of the lucky few who seem to have been born that way, it takes effort to achieve an optimistic, and happy outlook.

Most people prefer the path of least resistance. They are unwilling to make the changes that would give them a happier, more fulfilling life because it's just too much work. Besides, they believe change is scary. Better the devil you know than the one you don't.

WHEN CHANGE ISN'T SCARY, LIFE GETS HAPPY

Almost everything worth having in this life requires effort—effort to achieve in the first place, and more effort to maintain. If you think change is scary, try not changing! Fear can be useful when it helps us avoid danger. Generally, though, all it does is make us miserable and stops us from growing.

Dan Baker, a medical psychologist who has treated everyone from cardiac patients to people with eating disorders, believes that fear is the greatest enemy of happiness. In his book, *What Happy People Know* (Rodale, 2003; co-authored by Cameron Stauth), Baker says that fear of never having enough or never being enough keeps us unfulfilled and unhappy. I couldn't agree more. That's why *The Ten Principles* and this book focus on multiplying the positive aspects of your life. The more you can do that, the more you'll be able to bypass doubt and fear, and the happier you'll be.

"There's a powerful message in the thinking of positive psychology," says Robert J. Flynn, professor of psychology at the University of Ottawa. "It says we will not ignore people's limitations or weaknesses nor tried-and-true methods for dealing with them, but we will give equal time to developing their strengths and character. We're not all born optimists but we can learn to be that way."

When you are happy, you create a kind of emotional reservoir of positive feelings. If you regularly and genuinely appreciate what you receive from the people, animals and circumstances around you, you strengthen your "emotional immune system." You do this when you appreciate the past, too, by deliberately recalling memories of pleasant or poignant experiences.

The more you practice gratitude and appreciation, the more you will find that you have to appreciate. Whenever you practice anything, including responding positively to setbacks, no matter how you feel, you become more skillful at it. Then, the more skillful you are at practicing gratitude and banishing fear, the less power old negative patterns will have over you.

What's So Bad About Feeling Good?

Nothing at all—unless you're devoted to chasing "hit-and-run" happiness—you get a hit, and then it runs—unless you fail to do the things that lead to true and lasting satisfaction. In the case of hit-and-run Level One happiness, feeling good can become an obsession that causes excess—excess consumption, self-absorption, tension, and, ironically, excess loneliness and sadness. Life begins to feel out of balance.

In our culture, we are sold hit-and-run happiness every day, from a very young age. Many of the advertisements we see almost everywhere use our desire to feel good to sell us something—usually something we don't need. The ads often offer no information about their products. Instead, we see them worn or used within appealing contexts. We get the message: To feel good, we need to buy these things. Of course, they'll be outdated, unfashionable or obsolete soon, so we have to keep on buying, and buying, and buying.

Constantly running after transient, feel-good "fixes" is a recipe for spiritual disaster. Hit-and-run doesn't make you happy—for long, anyway. In fact, according to Dr. Martin Seligman, even "the cerebral virtues—curiosity and love of learning—are less likely to lead to happiness than interpersonal virtues, such as, kindness, gratitude and love."

THE MAGNIFICENT SEVEN

In Principle Nine, I outlined six practices that build self-esteem. Here are seven more practices that will help you build your happiness quotient.

1. **Gratitude.** Cultivate an appreciation for what you have. Learn to savor what you have created, earned or received as gifts. Say "thank you" often, and mean it.

2. **Simplicity.** The simpler your life, the easier it is to notice everyday joys. You will have more time to enjoy them. Try to simplify as much as possible.

3. **Health.** Treat your body with kindness and care, and it will reward you. Physical health and well-being should be among your top priorities.

4. **Compassion.** This may be the cardinal virtue. People who freely give and care about others tend to be happier, but you can't fake it. You have to practice.

5. **Persistence.** Almost everything that's needed to help you thrive is an acquired skill or belief. Acquisition means effort and time, patience and persistence.

6. **Acceptance.** Perfection isn't a prerequisite for happiness. Give the world permission to be okay just as it is, and give yourself permission to be human, and therefore, fallible.

7. **Support.** Fulfilling relationships are at the heart of happiness. When your human connections are

strong and supportive, you are more likely to thrive.

I call these seven practices *magnificent* for good reason. Value them as high priorities, incorporate them into your affirmations, make them part of your everyday consciousness, and see what happens to the quality of your life.

THE SPIRIT OF ENTELECHY
THE NEW POSITIVE PSYCHOLOGY

WHERE SCIENCE AND HAPPINESS MEET
Since the time of Socrates and Plato, "the good life" has been the subject of philosophical and religious inquiry. Psychology, a relatively modern science, has largely ignored the subject, focusing instead on understanding and remedying problems. As a result of this problem-centered focus, psychologists haven't spent much time studying the things that create happiness and make life worth living. Of course, their preoccupation with remedying human suffering should not be abandoned. Since both suffering and happiness are important parts of the human condition, we should be concerned with learning more about both.

Positive psychology is the scientific study of the strengths and virtues that enable individuals and communities to thrive. It aims to help people live and flourish rather than merely exist by discovering what does and doesn't work. This relates to: 1) Meeting life's challenges and making the most of setbacks and adversity, 2) engaging with and relating to other people, 3) finding fulfillment in creativity and productivity, and 4) looking beyond ourselves to help others find fulfillment and happiness.

Happiness is commonly defined as a state of well-being or pleasurable experience, but this notion of happiness is only a small part of positive psychology. Positive emotions lead to the pleasant life, which is one type of happiness. Using one's strengths in a challenging task leads to living a fully-engaged life, which creates another type of happiness. Using those strengths to serve something larger than yourself leads to yet another type of happiness—the deep and lasting kind created by a life of purpose and meaning.

POSITIVE PSYCHOLOGY AND POSITIVE THINKING

Positive thinking differs from positive psychology in two important ways. First, positive psychology is based on an empirical, replicable scientific study. Second, positive psychology recognizes that in spite of the many advantages of positive thinking, there are times when "realistic" or even negative thinking may be called for. Optimism and pessimism are complex concepts, although they are often portrayed in simple terms. Optimism is not *always* desirable, just as pessimism is not *always* undesirable.

Although studies show that optimism is associated with better health, improved performance, increased longevity and social success, there is evidence that in some situations negative thinking can produce more accuracy, which can sometimes have important consequences. For example, you would probably rather have your pilot or air traffic controller thinking realistically or even negatively rather than optimistically when deciding whether to approve takeoff during a severe ice storm.

It is also important to note that even positive thinking, which is usually a good and useful thing, can be taken to extremes. Human strengths are sometimes rooted in trial and *tribulation. Mastering difficulties tests our mettle, and boosts our self-esteem and self*-efficacy. Pushing ourselves to think only happy thoughts and have only happy experiences can limit our ability to think creatively and critically. Sometimes it is fine to settle for second best, and sometimes as the old country song says, we need to know when to "fold 'em."

We are all complex organisms, with a complete set of emotions. It is unrealistic to expect that we must always think or feel one way (positively) or always have only one kind of experience (successful or happy). Positive psychology's leading researchers are designing studies to learn more about what really does help us to flourish. The questions they are asking go far beyond the simplistic notion of, "Just think positively and all will be well," including the following:

- Does ignoring or downplaying *warranted* feelings of failure and anxiety really lead to happier, and more capable adults?

- Do children need to occasionally fail or feel sad/anxious/angry if they are to develop resiliency and experience success, joy and happiness?

- Do children need practice with the "three Ds" of dark, down, and disappointed as much as the more positive emotions?

- What about the "no day without night" argument? Does preventing bad feelings make it harder to know what feeling good is really like?

- Do some of the most successful and happy adults also have times that are filled with negative events? How did they develop the resilience to get past them?

WHAT POSITIVE PSYCHOLOGY KNOWS

Positive psychology researchers are discovering and confirming some things that might not be considered news. In fact, to many people they may seem like simple common sense. For starters:

- Wealth is only weakly related to happiness, particularly when income is above the poverty level.

- Activities that make people happy in small doses, such as shopping, good food and making money, do not lead to long-term fulfillment.

- A task or other experience that produces "flow" (absorption so great that you forget yourself and are fully "in the moment," with little or no awareness of time passing) is so gratifying that people will do it for its own sake. In other words, the activity is its own reward.

263

- People who often express gratitude are more optimistic, have better physical health, progress faster toward goals, have a greater sense of well-being, and tend to offer more help to others.

- Trying to maximize happiness in self-centered ways can lead to unhappiness.

- People who witness others performing good deeds experience emotions that motivate them to perform their own good deeds.

- Optimism can protect people from mental and physical illness.

- People who are happy or optimistic perform better at work, school, and on the playing field, are less depressed, have fewer health problems, and better relationships.

- People who report more positive emotions in young adulthood live longer and healthier lives.

- Physicians experiencing positive emotions tend to make more accurate diagnoses.

- Healthy human development can take place even under conditions of great adversity, due to a process of resilience that is common and completely ordinary.

- People are unable to accurately predict how long they will feel happy or sad following an important event. They typically overestimate how long they will be sad following a bad event, such as a romantic breakup, but fail to learn from repeated experiences that their predictions were wrong.

Do these research findings really add anything to what we already know? In fact, they do. They add certainty. It is easy to say something is obvious after the evidence is in, but the job of science is to prove or disprove what we assume to be true. Sometimes what we call common sense is valid, and sometimes it's not.

GOALS AND THE GOOD LIFE

If you are making more money these days but find that you are enjoying it less, you might want to re-examine and restructure your goals. If your happiness is based largely on Level One activities such as eating, earning or spending, yet you feel discontent, consider looking elsewhere for deeper, longer-lasting satisfaction. Find things to do that create flow, express more gratitude on a daily basis, and surround yourself with people who believe in selfless service. Set meaningful goals that will help you flourish as you never have before.

Not all goals are created equal. Your happiness and life satisfaction are profoundly influenced by goals to which you feel deeply committed, but when you doggedly strive for unattainable or foolish goals, it brings misery and suffering instead of joy and fulfillment. If your goals are largely focused on achieving fame and fortune, power or a successful image instead of intrinsically meaningful things like personal growth, harmonious relationships and community contribution, you are not likely to find deep or lasting happiness.

In fact, happiness is most often the result of activities that aren't about making you happy at all. That's why you need to know which of your goals are within reach, which you can grow into, which are not in your best interest, and, perhaps most importantly, which really matter. That's what the spirit of entelechy is all about.

What's more, positive psychologists tell us that avoidance goals—trying to steer clear of loneliness or things that upset you—don't have the same kind of positive outcomes as approach goals—trying to spend time with others or to stay calm in stressful circumstances. That is why *The Ten Principles* stresses that affirmations or goal statements must be written in approach rather than avoidance form. It is also why I emphasize eliminating negative self-talk.

SAVORING: A SKILL TO CELEBRATE

Even meaningful and manageable goals don't guarantee optimal life management. Assimilating the information in *The Ten Principles*, practicing persistently, and learning to appreciate and savor the blessings of the life you already have, will go a long way toward getting you there.

In 1995, the "Midlife in the United States" study surveyed a large representative sample of adults between the ages of twenty-five and seventy-four. Conducted by an interdisciplinary team of scholars and supported by the John D. and Catherine T. MacArthur Foundation, it found that fewer than two in ten adults were flourishing—that is, feeling and doing well on a daily basis. The study was widely reported in the press because it reflected something many, if not most, of us have felt. Our lives may be peaceful, and we may have material advantages undreamed of by our ancestors and much of the rest of the world, yet we continue to exist in a state of discontent. We don't savor our lives.

Savoring implies deliberately paying attention to the experience of pleasure. In other words, you choose to be aware, as fully as possible, of the things that make you happy, both when they happen and afterward. How do you learn to savor pleasure? Fred Bryant and Joseph Veroff of Loyola University detail five techniques you can borrow to promote savoring in your life.

1. **Share with others.** Tell other people about the experience and how much you value and enjoy it. The sooner the better.

2. **Build happy memories.** Take real life "mental" photographs of the experience or event, and revisit it later.

3. **Congratulate yourself.** If appropriate, remind yourself that you made this happen, how long you waited for it, how proud you are of yourself, and how proud others will be.

4. **Sharpen your perceptions.** Choose which parts of the experience you want to focus on and block out the others. Close your eyes while listening. Practice remembering details of color, taste, touch, and sound, etc.

5. **Immerse yourself.** Try not to think. Just feel or sense. Don't be distracted by other things you "should" be doing, wondering what will happen next, or how the experience could be ruined or improved upon. Be present in the present.

FINDING HAPPINESS THROUGH HARMONIOUS RELATIONSHIPS

Psychologists have a great deal to teach us about successful relationships of every kind, but particularly about intimate or love relationships. Dr. John Gottman, professor at the University of Washington and co-director of the Gottman Institute, is a groundbreaking, and widely respected marriage researcher. He can predict with more than 90 percent accuracy, which couples will stay together, and which will eventually divorce. He uses his knowledge to design programs that teach people how to change for the better. The six factors that most accurately predict divorce, according to Gottman, are these:

1. Harsh start-ups in disagreements

2. Criticism of one's partner rather than specific complaints

3. Expressions of contempt

4. Hair-trigger defensiveness

5. Lack of validation or stonewalling

6. Negative body language

Gottman can also predict which marriages will improve over the years. I had to learn these things the hard way. I learned from Darcy. It all emanated from unshakable commitment to improving. Here are the relatively simple things that Gottman says these couples do—practices that are perfectly compatible with *The Ten Principles* and which I highly recommend.

Take a minute or two to ask what your partner is going to do that day before you say good-bye in the morning. Take another few minutes for a low-stress "reunion" conversation at the end of the day. Add plenty of affection (touching, holding, kissing, and sweet talk), throw in a weekly "date" in a relaxed atmosphere, and top it off with at least one expression of admiration or appreciation every day.

BLESSED WITH A PURPOSE

In the course of my work, I talk with many people who are committed to professions or personal endeavors that they never consciously planned to pursue. Some say they feel trapped. Often, they attribute the direction their lives have taken to chance or circumstance. They have been forced, they believe, to take on roles they don't enjoy but must tolerate.

Positive psychology researchers tell us that a strong sense of purpose enhances overall contentment. I believe that each of us has been blessed with a purpose, and our mission is to discover it. I also believe that striving to discover your purpose and life's work can help you realize your true potential to live a more authentic, and satisfying life. It's never too late to start.to discover your purpose, consider your interests in the present and the passions that moved you in the past. Perhaps you felt attracted to a certain profession when you were young, but veered away from it for so-called practical reasons. Or perhaps you have an interest that is largely unexplored. What calls to you? What sort of work gets you excited? You may well discover your life's work within the context of your current occupation. If you want to change the world, could you continue doing what you do for a different kind of employer or organization? If you're not sure where to begin, assessing your beliefs, strengths, passions and values is a good place to start your quest for purpose. Create affirmations to support your search and visualize them daily.

Since any lifelong journey is one of evolution, you may need to redefine your direction from time to time. For instance, being an amazing parent can be your principal purpose for eighteen years. Then you may want different work to do. Remember, your life's work may not be something you are recognized or financially compensated for, such as parenting, a beloved hobby, or a variety of other activities others may deem inconsequential. Your love for a pursuit is what gives it meaning. You will know that you have discovered your life's work when you wake up eager to face each day and find yourself feeling good, not only about what you do, but also about who you are.

The Spirit of Entelechy
Self-Assessment and Transformation

What Don't You Like?

What if you could take everything you're currently dissatisfied with and resolve it? A life without frustration or dissatisfaction—can you imagine such a thing?

I hope you can, because if you are willing to do what it takes, you can deal with your frustrations and dissatisfactions in ways that will help you grow, bring you pleasure, or both. Here's how.

List ten or twelve things you don't like about your life, in no particular order. Be complete, honest and brief. Here's a sample list.

I don't like:

- getting up at 6:00 a.m.

- feeling lonely so much

- that my house is so messy

- how unattractive my teeth look

- how angry I get at my kids

- making cold calls

- the extra twenty pounds I have put on

- that I don't excel at anything

- my escalating stress level

- my neighborhood

- not having enough money

- my father's new wife

After you've made your list, check each statement below that describes your current reality.

I feel bored too often.

I could accomplish a lot more than I do.

I am stuck in a rut.

There is little or no passion or purpose in my life.

I am just going through the motions at work.

I do too much "magical thinking" (things will work out well, even though I do little or nothing to see that they do).

I feel lonely too much. I don't enjoy my own company.

My finances are a mess.

Some of my relationships are a mess.

My house is a mess.

Most of the time, I don't take good care of myself.

I distract myself so I don't have to deal with problems.

GET YOUR PRIORITIES STRAIGHT

Rate each item on your list and each checked statement with either a 1 = strong dislike, and very disruptive, or a 2 = milder dislike, and less disruptive. From the #1 group, choose the one that is most upsetting. In case of a tie, flip a coin. From the #2 group, choose the one that seems easiest to remedy. If you're not certain, just take your best guess.

You are about to tackle these two items, but don't throw the list away. The process of creating it should have raised your consciousness a bit. Making progress on two of your dissatisfactions will shore up your self-esteem and sense of personal power, so you probably won't want to stop there.

Turn Gripes Into Goals

The following three-step plan may seem too simple to be effective, but don't be deceived. It works—there's no question about that—but it also takes work. You need to plan that work and work the plan. If you leave out even one step, you will strip the process of its power.

1. **Affirm and visualize**. First, review Principle Eight, which is all about why affirmations work and how to write them. Then, using the present tense, write a sentence that vividly describes how it will look (sound, smell, taste, etc.) and, most importantly, how you will feel when the situation has been positively and permanently resolved. Remember, you can't affirm change in anyone but yourself. Repeat this step for each item or area you have chosen to work on.

   Spend five minutes a day, morning and night, visualizing these two affirmations. Pay particular attention to generating and experiencing the positive feelings that accompany them.

2. **Change your behavior to support your affirmations.** This is key. You can affirm and visualize until the cows come home, but if your behavior doesn't change, little else will either, except maybe your position on the couch. For each item or area you're working on, list several specific, *quantifiable* changes you intend to make in your own behavior or attitude to improve the situation.

   This is where the rubber meets the road. Transitions are notoriously tough, especially when they involve tough problems, so don't be surprised by stress. Used creatively, stress can stoke rather than zap energy, but it can still take a toll. It's old news, but bears repeating—get enough rest and if you don't already exercise, start. Take good care of your body and it will reward you.

3. **Believe in your ability to grow into your vision.** Map out a plan and follow it. Measure your progress and adjust the plan if needed. That's all there is to it, except for patience and persistence. Great leaps of progress are rare, although they do happen. More commonly, though, we grow and change incrementally. Moving forward toward the life you want little by little will get you there, so don't quit. Enlist support along the way. Try it on the first two items, congratulate/reward yourself, and then tackle the rest. It works. What are you waiting for?

THE SPIRIT OF ENTELECHY
HIGH-LEVEL LIVING

HABITUAL HIGH-LEVEL LIVING

In Principle Ten, I described many benefits and advantages of Level Three and Level Four thinking. What do you do if you really want to move toward the deep and long-lasting kind of happiness that these levels bring? You are serious about maximizing the good you can do with your talents and skills. You want to look for and find the good in others, not only for your sake and theirs, but also for the sake of generations to come—but how do you make these very desirable, high-level behaviors become natural and normal?

The process may not be easy, but what you've learned from *The Ten Principles* will help enormously. While your conscious mind is saying, "Yes, I absolutely do want to change so I can realize the benefits of Level Three living," it is likely that your subconscious is saying, "No way. I'm not sure that being different will be a good thing, and change is uncomfortable, so I'll stay the way I am."

Even so, you can consciously choose to stop being a house divided. A clear vision of what you want together with the three P's—practice, patience and persistence—will generate new behavior, again and again. Eventually, it will eclipse the old and become second nature—a new habit.

Sure, your old ways and your new intentions will be in conflict for a while. Expect it. When you have a vision for positive change and you are trying your best to build a new habit, there are normally some ups and downs, and some tension and stress. Remember the cognitive dissonance I talked about in Principle Seven? It's a predictable part of wanting something new and being dissatisfied with the old. If you stick with your efforts, though, before long you will arrive at a place where you feel more comfortable with the new you than you ever did with the old. Much of the stress of change will have worn off. In its place will be a wonderful new clarity and confidence.

That doesn't mean you're home free. Relapse and regression are still hazards, and setbacks can be particularly hard to take at this point, but *The Ten Principles* offer many tools you can use in dealing with them. As always, the sooner you pick yourself up, dust yourself off and get back on track again, the better. You don't have to start all over at square one, either. Just pick up where you left off and keep going.

After Level Three thinking starts to feel like second nature, you'll find yourself with a tremendous new supply of energy and enthusiasm. Since there is no longer an internal struggle (I can/I can't; I am/I'm not), you will also find yourself enjoying a new sense of calm and contentment.

Of course, relapse is still possible, especially during times when you're feeling fatigued, experiencing sudden or dramatic change, or under high stress. If that happens, take it easy on yourself and those around you. Keep your goal uppermost in mind, control your self-talk, and affirm your resiliency at the same time you continue to affirm the desired end-result.

Four Level Three Pitfalls

As with so many other potentially beneficial activities, a Level Three attitude can sometimes shift into a less benevolent state. It can even become downright dangerous. If you become ensnared in any of the following attitudinal traps, you may find yourself back in Level One or Level Two behaviors before you realize it. Be sure to monitor yourself, and avoid:

1. **The comparison contest.** Try not to compare your behavior with others. If it doesn't make you feel bad because you know you're not doing as much as some people are, you may end up congratulating yourself, which is, in some ways, even worse. If you think what you are doing is better (more effective, widespread,

useful, selfless, etc.) than what someone else is doing, you've already fallen back to Level Two thinking. Don't go there.

2. **The judgment jeopardy.** Do you try to help others improve by pointing out what they're doing wrong or criticizing them "for their own good?" Are you sure they'd be better off if they would only listen? Do you give unasked-for advice or try to pressure others into growth? This harms relationships. It makes it hard for people to trust you or for you to trust them, and it makes your good intentions moot. It works against happiness all around. Don't go there, either.

3. **The burnout bailout.** Do you know people who always seem to be doing something for a good cause? They can't seem to get enough service to others crammed into their lives. They enjoy it so much or they feel so driven that they end up doing too much. They can't say no, feel overwhelmed and exhausted as a result, and eventually burn out. To avoid the pitfall of burnout, which invites low-level thinking and bad feelings, make *focus and prioritizing* your mantra.

4. **The savior stall.** If you believe everything depends on you, you're in trouble. You can't relax, don't rest enough, your energy is spent keeping things together, putting out fires, and tending to the big picture as well as the details. This makes you a prime candidate for burnout, one of the least productive states you can spend time in. If you don't burn out, you will end up forcing others to depend on you to such an extent that your ability to support them will eventually be compromised.

Sometimes, if they see you falling into one of these traps, the people close to you will say something. Don't count on it. Depending on how they think, you are likely to respond, "And what else is going on in your life?" They may simply choose to avoid you, ignore you, get angry with you or sabotage you. Don't wait for a wake-up call from the outside world.

Instead, take time to reflect and recharge, and do it regularly. Schedule it, as you would anything else important. Reserve as much time as you need and approach it with an open mind, pen or keyboard in hand. Consider asking for candid feedback from people you trust, or allow them to make it anonymously. Pay attention to what they have to say. Stop yourself before you sabotage your own efforts.

At Level Four, I talk about ultimate good, and ultimate purpose. These are lofty words, and they have their own pitfalls. Striving for the ultimate can lead to expectations that are unrealistically high. You can't get ultimate happiness or love, ultimate purpose or meaning, from other people, organizations, or even from causes. Remember, life at Levels Three and Four isn't about "getting" anything. It's all about giving. Ultimate experiences, by definition, leave no room for growth or development. They can only be had in an ultimate realm—the realm of spiritual connection, however you define spirit.

TAKE A LEAP OF FAITH

If you find yourself wanting something that seems outrageous or unattainable such as living your life on Level Three, it may feel like standing at the edge of a precipice, looking out over the abyss at your vision. Do you resist the urge to jump, feeling paralyzed by the gap between current circumstances and the life of your dreams? Or do you choose to take a leap of faith into the unknown, unsure of what you will encounter there, but certain that you could gain more in your attempt than by giving in to your fearful, self-protective instincts?

Taking a leap of faith can be exceedingly difficult, especially for people with control issues. This, as Darcy often points out, includes just about everyone. The act of embracing uncertainty means you must trust that your efforts will net you the rewards you seek. I believe, based on experience and research studies, that such trust is justified. When you take a leap of faith, believing without a doubt that you will land safely on the other side, you can accomplish almost anything you set out to do.

A successful leap of faith requires your attention, as it is the quiet and often indistinct voice of your inner self that will point you toward your ultimate destination. When you see that arriving at your destination means you must step outside of the boundaries of established comfort zones and jettison yourself into a new phase of your life, thinking about taking that plunge can be scary. While you may fear what seems to be an inevitable fall, in all likelihood, you will find yourself flying.

It's true that the leap across the chasm of ambiguity may challenge you in unforeseen, and unpredictable ways. Trust yourself. You will make it across. If your mind and heart are apprehensive and stubbornly resist, build a bridge of knowledge. The more you know about the leap you're poised to take, the smaller the gap becomes between "here" and "there." Then it will appear be easier for you to let go of the old and embrace the new.

Your courageous leap of faith can lead you into uncharted territory, enabling you to build a new, more adventurous, and meaningful life. Though you may anticipate that fear will be your guide on your journey across the abyss, you will likely discover that it is exhilaration and excitement that become your constant companions.

Why Bother?

Why would you, or anyone else, want to go to all the trouble, all the effort, and all the disruption of the status quo, to change their ways of thinking and behaving and move to Level Three, let alone Level Four?

The answer is simple:

- You do it to live a purpose-driven life that is truly worth living.

- You do it so that your ability to do well and find lasting happiness will be maximized.

- You do it so that on the day you die, and on every day before it, you will have no regrets.

When you serve a greater cause—along with your talents and skills—you bring goodness to everything you do. You begin to live, not merely exist, and live in a way that truly satisfies.

Moreover, it feels good to do well. You become more energized, more creative, and more open to possibility—even more humorous. It is easy to laugh at yourself and at the follies and foibles of the world when your heart is filled with kindness and compassion instead of anxiety and self-interest. Of course, your relationships are vastly improved by this attitude—at work, at home, and everywhere you go. By looking for the good in others, you will discover more good in yourself.

Striving to live on Level Three doesn't mean you never again experience fear, anger, resentment, self-pity, discouragement, and all the other so-called negative emotions. When you control your self-talk and bring the same love and compassion you show others to yourself, they are short-lived. Like the good you do, the work you do on yourself is never wasted.

Remember, the longer happiness lasts, the better it is. The more widespread happiness is, the better it is. The deeper happiness is, the better it is. When you deliberately and thoughtfully choose the levels of happiness you want to experience, your time on earth becomes much richer. When you enlarge and expand your vision of who you can be, what you can contribute, and how you'll go about realizing your dreams, you will live a meaningful, and happier life.

THE SPIRIT OF ENTELECHY

PERSONAL ETHICS

EVERYDAY ETHICS

"Have you taken the mandatory training for business ethics?" Dilbert's manager asked the popular comic strip engineer one day. Without missing a beat, Dilbert turns from his cubicle's computer and responds, "No, but if you say I did, then you'll save some money on training, which you can spend to decorate your office." Obviously taken with this suggestion, the manager says, "Luckily, I haven't taken the training myself." Dilbert adds, "I hear it's mostly common sense anyway." The ethics Dilbert is talking about might be called everyday or personal ethics.

Ethics involves standards of conduct. These standards define how we should behave, based on moral duties and virtues, which themselves come from standards based on accepted ideas of right and wrong. The terms "values" and "ethics" are similar, but not interchangeable. Ethics is concerned with how a moral person should behave, whereas values are simply the beliefs and attitudes that determine how we actually do behave. Clearly, on that day, what Dilbert and his manager valued most had nothing to do with ethics.

While we must all decide for ourselves what our moral obligations are, to say that ethics are "personal" may be slightly misleading. An individual's conscience generally includes a wider range of values and beliefs than do universal ethical norms. When personal values supplement accepted ethical norms with moral convictions, there is no conflict. Unfortunately, some people try to impose their personal moral judgments on others as if they were universal ethical norms.

Others adopt personal codes of conduct that are inconsistent with universal ethical norms. Clearly, not all choices and value systems, however dearly held, are equally ethical. If they were, there would be no legitimate basis for distinguishing between Hitler and Gandhi.

A person who believes that certain races are inferior to others, and therefore that it is "right" to oppress or persecute those races, has adopted a personal value system that is inherently unethical. Similarly, someone who has decided that lying is okay if it is done to achieve an important personal goal is not behaving ethically.

We all have the right to choose our own values, but all choices and value systems do not have an equal right to be called ethical. When I talk about personal ethics in this chapter, I simply mean ethics in your personal life, away from the workplace. Of course, you can't have one set of ethics for home and another set to use at work. Since we have already addressed professional issues in Part III, I will discuss the personal aspect of ethical behavior separately here.

ETHICAL COMMITMENT

Ethical commitment is a strong desire to do the right thing, even if it means we have to pay financial, social or emotional costs. Surveys reveal that regardless of profession, almost all of us believe that we are, or should be, ethical. While most of us say we are not satisfied with the ethical quality of society as a whole, we believe that our profession is more ethical than others, and that we are at least as ethical as others in our profession. Unfortunately, behavior does not consistently conform to self-image and moral ambitions. As a result, a substantial number of decent people who feel committed to ethical values regularly compromise these values, often because they lack the courage to follow their conscience.

Ethical principles should be seen as the ground rules of our decision-making process, not just factors to consider. We need to remember that it is okay to lose. In fact, it is better to lose than to lie, steal, or cheat in order to win. If you are not willing to lose now and then, it means you have to be willing to do whatever it takes to win, even if that means abandoning your ethical principles. Being ethical has a price. *Sometimes people have to choose between what they want and who they want to be.*

Ethics also has a value, which makes self-restraint and sacrifice, service and charity, deeply and completely worthwhile.

YOUR PERSONAL CODE OF ETHICS

I highly recommend that you develop your own code of ethics, rather than relying on what others have taught you or expect of you. This doesn't diminish the fact that you may have had some wonderful teachers in your life, but until you investigate, take ownership and internalize your own code of ethics, you will never truly be the master of your heart, mind and soul.

A personal code of ethics defines the ideas about right and wrong that are the essence of your life. It is a written document that allows you to say, "I will do this because I believe this," and serves not only as a reminder of what you believe, but also as an encouragement to carry on with your quest for a Level Three life. Here's how to create one.

1. **Take a personal inventory.**

Who are you? What character traits involving morality do you most value in yourself? What are your virtues? What kind of person are you striving to become? If you asked a dear friend or loving parent to describe you, what would they say? Write it all down. Don't worry about sounding "full of yourself." Be honest.

What do you believe? List your beliefs that involve ethical or moral behavior. Don't worry about why you believe them; just write down as many as you can call to mind. Start with the sentence stem, "I believe people should…" and complete the sentence as many times as you can.

Why do you believe this? This is an important part of the process because it helps you more fully own and understand your beliefs. The source of many ethical beliefs is a religious text, so if you have favorite Bible or Koran verses, note them next to the appropriate belief. Perhaps the source is a philosopher, teacher, parent or grandparent. Again, write them down.

2. **Draft your code of ethics.** This isn't as difficult as it might seem at first, though it requires a bit of time and energy. Consider carefully what you want to include.

The first part defines the purpose of your code. Why do you want it? Are you creating it to correct your behavior or to inspire you to greater heights? What's your goal? Make this as personal as possible—not what you think will look or sound good, but your real reasons.

The second part lists the rules or beliefs you expect yourself to follow when dealing with other people. These should encompass the beliefs and reasons you listed in your inventory. Try using the sentence stem, "I will…" and complete the sentence as many times as you wish, until you think you have all the bases covered.

After you have finished the first draft, put it aside for a day or two. Then take it out again and look it over. Refine it as necessary or as situations in your life bring new ethical aspects to light.

3. **Live by your code.** When you are confronted with a moral or ethical decision, your belief system will be put to the test. If there's time, get out your code and review it. It is there to guide you and remind you of what matters, so use it. Don't allow yourself to be pressured into violating your code. Don't rationalize your violations, either. Ask anyone who has ever behaved unethically why they did it, and they will likely have no trouble citing what they considered "good" reasons. The end doesn't justify the means, and you don't want to fall into that ultimately self-destructive trap.

Self-awareness is key. Avoid reacting in a knee-jerk way through habit or prejudice. Instead, take time to try to perceive the right and wrong in a situation. Think through the consequences, and use your code of ethics to help you consciously choose the right alternative. Develop your ability to connect cause and effect, as well. Practice seeing the things that happen to you as the result of earlier actions performed by you, not as random events, and stop seeing yourself as a victim. When you do this, you will become master of your destiny, proactively creating the future you want by choosing to behave in ways that are most likely to cause it.

THE SPIRIT OF ENTELECHY
THE POWER OF A SMILE

BELIEFS DRIVE BEHAVIOR, AND BEHAVIOR SHAPES BELIEFS

Perhaps the most effective way to change the quality of your life is to change your beliefs. Changed behavior automatically follows, and changed behavior creates new results. For example, if you believe that people are not to be trusted, your behavior will be defensive. Defensive behavior usually elicits a similar response, which you will interpret as evidence that your belief is well-founded. On the other hand, if you believe that people are trustworthy, you'll approach them with a friendly, open spirit, provoking friendliness from them, and once again, confirm your belief.

This process is called a self-fulfilling prophecy, and it happens all the time. We get back mostly what we give. We see mostly what we expect to see, and our beliefs are generally confirmed by our experiences, because our beliefs *create* our experiences.

Another way to change the quality of your life is to start with behavior. See what happens when you *act as if: as if* you were a friendly, outgoing person; a*s if* you were confident and caring, patient and kind; *as if* you were a positive force for good in the world; *as if* you were already all the things you would most like to be; as *if* you were living a Level Three life; and *as if* you were genuinely happy. Of course, if you really want to speed up the change process, I recommend you do both—work on changing your beliefs and your behavior at the same time.

Happiness Creates Success

Conventional wisdom says that people become happy as a result of a number of external conditions—because they are healthy, are held in high esteem by their peers, feel powerful and competent, have a good marriage, or have a large and growing bank account. Studies conducted at several U.S. universities during the last few years tell us it's really the other way around. Most people aren't happy because they are successful—they are successful because they are happy.

That shouldn't surprise us. Happy people are usually easier to work with and be around (although if they're inappropriately cheerful they can be pretty annoying). They are more highly motivated and willing to tackle difficult projects, so it's no wonder they are more likely to succeed.

Add a Little Now To Your Later

Happiness is most likely to descend upon us, says psychologist Lee Jampolsky, "When we are able to adopt an outlook on life where we stop seeing the outside world as the determiner of our happiness, and instead, see our thoughts as the determiner of happiness. It's about changing our thoughts."

Dr. Jampolsky, author of, *Smile for No Good Reason*, says that one of the key things you can do to be happy is, "Add a little now to your later." He explains that, "If you're only worrying about the future, it's very difficult to be happy. It's in the present moment that we find our sense of happiness and peace." To help yourself be more "present in the present," why not affirm and visualize it? *The time for me to be happy is now.* Write it on a Post-it note and stick it on your bathroom mirror, dashboard, computer monitor, or cubicle wall.

Humor as Healer

Although used throughout history, interest in humor as a healing agent probably originated in the 1970s, when Norman Cousins, editor of *The Saturday Review,* detailed his experiences in *Anatomy of an Illness* and *The Healing Heart.* According to his own accounts, Cousins overcame a potentially fatal chronic disease by laughing at favorite comedy shows. He said that ten minutes of laughing gave him two hours of drug-free pain relief. Later, he helped himself recover from a serious heart attack using the same method. At the time, many people considered Cousins a crackpot. Since then, many research studies have supported his ideas, showing that laughing can indeed help us heal by:

- lowering blood pressure

- reducing stress hormones

- increasing muscle flexion

- boosting immune functions by raising levels of infection-fighting T-cells, disease-fighting proteins and disease-destroying antibodies

- triggering the release of endorphins—the body's natural painkillers

- producing a general sense of well-being.

About fifteen years ago, an Indian physician and yoga student created a practice called Laughter Yoga. Thanks to him, there are now more than 5,000 "laughter clubs" in more than fifty countries. The laughter exercises he recommends almost always lead to real laughter, especially when practiced in a group.

Hey U.G.L.Y (Unique Gifted Lovable You—www.heyugly.com) is a wonderful nonprofit organization dedicated to helping teens boost their self-esteem. They have created a CD called *Laugh It Off*, which consists mainly of sixty minutes of real laughter on an audio track. You are supposed to follow along for a while, laughing. I tried it and could not stop grinning!

These are just three examples, yet there are countless others. Look for reasons to laugh, or just do it for no reason at all. Daily doses of laughter may turn out to be, as *The Reader's Digest* has claimed for decades, the best medicine.

START WITH A SMILE
Can we really control our own level of happiness? Although we all have genetic predispositions, genes are not the sold determinants of a happy

disposition. I am convinced that all of us have more control over our moods than we may think. If you want to be happier, what better place to start than with a smile?

Unless you're a psychologist, you have probably never heard of "facial feedback," a theory that says feedback from our facial expressions provides neural stimulation that affects our emotions. In plain English, this means that you can probably improve your mood just by smiling! When you smile, you release more serotonin and endorphins, the "happiness hormones," which boost your energy, strengthen your immune system, and reduce any stress or pain you may be feeling.

It doesn't stop there. When you smile, you are likely to improve other people's moods, too. No doubt you know this from your own experience. You're having a bad day when out of the blue, someone gives you a million kilowatt smile—doesn't matter who, doesn't matter if you know them or not, either. Suddenly, your spirits lift. If you return the smile, as is likely, your mood lifts even more. Then why wait for "out of the blue?" Why not be the one who makes it happen?

JUST FOR TODAY, SMILE AT IT
In *The Ten Principles* seminar, we ask participants to eliminate negative self-talk for twenty-four hours, as a consciousness raiser. The results are always amazing. Here's another radical idea. For twenty-four hours, smile at much as possible—at other people and as a response to things that happen to you. Your smile may be amused, bemused or even confused. Sometimes it will be delighted, sometimes surprised, or perhaps it will be a smile of love or compassion. Aim to make every smile, no matter what kind it is or what the circumstance may be, a smile that expresses genuine pleasure. Of course, that means you must find something to be pleased about in every circumstance. Make sure it doesn't stop at your mouth; a real smile always reaches the eyes.

You don't need a reason to smile beyond choosing to, and the "whatever" that happens to you doesn't have to be good. Just for a day, try smiling, simply as a matter of course. Being alive and kicking is reason enough, if you think about it. Don't worry about turning into one of those smiley emoticons or looking like an idiot, either. If you weren't one to start with, that won't be a problem. You are likely to turn into a person who feels and makes others happier.

HAVING TROUBLE FINDING A SMILE?
Try one of these:

- Jump on the bed (my personal favorite, not Darcy's!)

- Make faces at yourself in the mirror

- Dance to wild and crazy music

- Go to a playground and watch, or better yet, play

- Give someone you love a bear hug

- Watch some cartoons you loved as a kid

- Rent videos of zany TV shows: Scrubs, Friends, or Seinfeld

- Rent videos of whacky movies—Peter Sellers, Adam Sandler, or Ben Stiller

- Visit a pet store; pet the puppies

- Have a pillow fight with a family member, not necessarily a kid

THE SPIRIT OF ENTELECHY
EVERYDAY PHILANTHROPY

EVERYONE HAS SOMETHING TO OFFER
Many people think that philanthropy is only for the wealthy. Not so. Maybe if we get rid of the fancy language and call it what it really is—giving to charity—it will be easier to take to your heart. Everyday philanthropy is any kind of giving that happens on a regular basis and is intended to serve the greater good. It can be an important and rewarding part of life, especially for those of us who want to spend more time on Level Three.

No matter what your income, no matter what your circumstances, you and your family members can be philanthropists, making a positive difference in the world. Alec Dickson, the late founder of the British volunteer service after which John Kennedy modeled our Peace Corps, was fond of saying that you don't necessarily need a big solution to solve a big problem; many small, individual actions added together can change the world.

TEACHING KIDS TO GIVE
One of the greatest gifts parents can give children is a sense of involvement in their community, so include them in philanthropic activities. Ask everyone for input when choosing projects and researching charitable organizations, and ask your kids about their personal priorities and interests.

Kids learn by example, so it's up to you to show them the way. If you and your children explore the world of philanthropy side-by-side, you'll be helping them see how what they do or don't do impacts the world.

Make giving part of your everyday life by setting up a family philanthropy fund. This doesn't have to involve a lot of money—collecting spare change once a week can mount up and make a difference. If your kids earmark part of their allowance for charity from an early age, and you make sure they see where it's going and how it's helping others, personal responsibility and global citizenship is likely to become second nature to them.

THE LADDER OF GIVING

Maimonides, a twelfth century scholar, invented the following ladder of giving. Each rung represents a higher degree of virtue.

1. Giving begrudgingly, making the recipient feel disgraced or embarrassed.

2. Giving cheerfully, but giving too little.

3. Giving cheerfully and adequately, but only after being asked.

4. Giving without being asked.

5. Giving when you don't know the recipient, but the recipient knows who you are.

6. Giving when you know the recipient, but the recipient doesn't know who you are.

7. Giving when neither you nor the recipient knows the other's identity.

8. The highest: Giving money, a loan, your time or whatever it takes to help someone become more self-reliant.

WHAT TO GIVE AND WHO TO GIVE TO

Imagine how the world would change if we all rose even to Level 4—giving before being asked! There are so many ways to support charitable causes and make a real difference in one life, a community, or in the world. These are some of the most common:

- Donate money

- Volunteer time

- Donate usable goods instead of tossing them away

- Organize or participate in charity auctions

- Organize or participate in sports events for charity

- Give routinely—buy a few extra non-perishables at the grocery store and leave them in the food bank barrel; give repeatedly to those who "are always out there" soliciting donations for a cause you support.

If you haven't been a regular volunteer in the past, you may be perplexed about finding something that fits your personality. Here's a list to help you find the perfect match.

HOMELESS SHELTERS
Almost all homeless shelters need volunteers to help prepare or distribute meals, work in the office, organize a food drive to stock the pantry, collect clothing for shelter residents, or deliver brown-bag lunches to the homeless.

FOOD BANK
Food banks often work with shelters, but they also serve poor people in the community, especially around the holidays. You could collect food, help manage inventory, or distribute food to those in need.

CHILDREN'S WISHES
The Children's Wish Foundation is a nonprofit dedicated to bringing joy and hope to seriously ill kids through the magic of a fulfilled wish. Refer a child, volunteer your time, or help make a wish come true.

PARKS AND OUTDOOR AREAS
Most city and state parks have volunteer programs. You can assist with educational programs, trail construction/maintenance, pick up/clean up trash, plant flowers, shrubs, or trees.

LITERACY AND LEARNING

Too many adults have never learned to read or read at a grade school level. Literacy volunteers help kids and adults learn this important skill. Prisons and jails need literacy programs, as well. Become a tutor, work in the office, or collect books to donate to libraries, prisons, jails, and shelters.

TUTORING AND MENTORING

The limited resources of many public schools, especially those in inner-city areas, means inadequate education for too many kids. Children in shelters need extra help, as they have probably missed a lot of school due to circumstances out of their control. You can be a tutor, classroom contact or online e-mail buddy.

SAVE THE PLANET

Many environmental groups encourage volunteer support. Help lobby on conservation issues, lead educational hikes and other activities, lend a hand at the office, start a Reuse, Reduce and Recycle campaign, or ask your local recycling center if they have a project they could use help with.

ANIMAL WELFARE

Volunteer at PAWS or your local humane society. Walk dogs, socialize cats, help with fundraising, animal welfare education or adoptions, keep facilities clean or assist with general office support.

SPECIAL OLYMPICS

The Special Olympics is an international program of year-round sports training and competition for children and adults with developmental disabilities. They offer a number of volunteer activities, including sports training, administrative help, competition planning or staffing. What a great way to make others feel special!

BUILD HOMES
Habitat for Humanity builds and donates houses to poor people in local communities all over the country. Their volunteers learn a lot about hands-on construction techniques and perform a great service.

HOSPITALS
Almost all hospitals have volunteer programs to help patients both inside and outside the wards. Contact several local hospitals to learn more.

LIBRARIES
Many libraries need help re-shelving books, running children's programs, receiving and cataloging donations, and making books available to the community. Call your local branch and ask about volunteer opportunities.

SENIOR CITIZENS
Most senior centers need volunteers to provide companionship and activities to seniors. Call one and see what kinds of programs they have. You could do house or yard work at an elderly person's home, play chess or checkers with an elder, teach classes or lead group activities.

CITY PROGRAMS
Call around to see what volunteer opportunities are available where you live. You might brighten a public play area or inner-city building with a mural, paint swing sets in bright colors at a playground, place wood chips, and create slide landings.

BLOOD BANKS
There are volunteer opportunities in most blood banks across the country. Find a local blood bank in the phone book or online and see what you can do to help.

DISASTER RELIEF
Volunteers are extremely vital during times of disaster, and there is always a disaster of some sort in some place on the globe. The Red

Cross, Mercy Corps, and other relief organizations are usually happy to have help. Give them a call and ask what you can do to support them, in addition to giving cash.

POLITICAL CAMPAIGNS

If it's an election year, there are countless opportunities to volunteer, no matter where you live. Pick a candidate whose ideas you believe in on the local, state or national level and volunteer to be a part of the campaign.

HOTLINES

Many crisis clinics or 1-800 help lines rely on volunteers to answer phones and handle other tasks. If there's an 800-phone bank or crisis line in your area, they will be happy to have your help.

BOYS AND GIRLS CLUBS

Local YMCAs/YWCAs and Boys and Girls Clubs always offer volunteer opportunities ranging from childcare to coaching. Check with their volunteer coordinators for more information.

MUSEUMS

Museums are wonderful places to volunteer, especially if you love art, science or history. Docents and tour guides meet lots of people and help them better understand and appreciate what they're seeing. Contact any museum (art, sculpture, science, children's) in your area to learn more.

Giving is a vital part of the spirit of entelechy, Level-Three living, and of developing fully as a human being. Make everyday philanthropy part of your everyday life. It will make you a better person and the world a better place.

THE SPIRIT OF ENTELECHY

SPIRIT IN LOVE

WHAT'S LOVE GOT TO DO WITH IT?

The word *love* is derived from the Sanskrit lubh (to desire) and Latin lubere (to please). But does love describe a feeling, a way of behaving, or both? Some people say love is mysterious, magical and indefinable. Others try to look more closely.

John Gray, author of the best-selling Mars and Venus series of books, defines love as, "A feeling directed at someone which acknowledges their goodness." M. Scott Peck, author of what is perhaps the clipper ship of self-help books, *The Road Less Traveled,* says love is more than a feeling. Peck describes love as, "The willful intent to serve the well-being of another." Going even further, The Bible's book of Corinthians tells us that love is patient and kind, does not envy or boast, is not proud, rude, or self-seeking, is not easily angered and keeps no record of wrongs. It always protects, trusts, hopes and perseveres. Is this a tall order—too lofty for most of us to fill? Or is it a noble and achievable aspiration, based on the truth of our essential nature?

There is probably no part of our lives in which spirit is felt, tested, and rewarded more than in our love relationships. The people we love and by whom we are loved, particularly our husbands, wives and sweethearts, are all too often the people we wound and are wounded by. Love asks us to be vulnerable. It also asks us to forgive and forget, over and over again. As such, if we honor it and stick with it, love can usher us into a place where our spirit expands and overflows with generosity and goodness. In this place, Level Three relationships are not only possible, they are the norm.

TEN WAYS TO PUT MORE LOVE IN YOUR LIFE

1. **Cultivate the attitude of gratitude.** As the old song advises, count your blessings instead of sheep when you go to sleep. Keep a gratitude journal. Say thank you for something specific to your partner at least once a day. Put some of your thank you's in writing—cards, letters, and sticky notes on the fridge.

2. **Arrange regular solo time.** Schedule time to reflect, recharge, and relax. Remember what you value, who you are, and who you want to be. Encourage your partner to do the same. Support each other's efforts to find solo time with childcare, taking on more household tasks, and gentle reminders, etc.

3. **Be good to yourself.** This ought to go without saying—unfortunately, it doesn't. Take care of yourself! Commit random acts of self-nurturing and sensible acts of self-love on a daily basis. Don't expect to get from others what you are unwilling to give to yourself.

4. **Slow down and simplify.** If your life is over-busy, your to-do list endless, and your calendar filled weeks in advance, it's a safe bet that your relationship is suffering. Look at your Balance Wheel again and get your priorities straight.

5. **Smile more.** Mother Teresa was once asked how to make the world a better place if you couldn't dedicate your life to helping the poor. She said, "Smile more." Smile at your partner twice as much as you do now. Start the smile in your heart, and then bring it up into your mouth and eyes. This is transformative.

6. **Look for the good and praise it.** Tell your partner what you like, admire, and find attractive about him/her. Do it often. If you try, you can find something favorably to comment about every day. Don't assume

he/she already knows, and shouldn't have to be told. It doesn't work that way.

7. **Touch and be touched.** Human beings need to be touched. When you put plenty of affectionate touching into your relationship, it and you are more likely to thrive.

8. **Look through the eyes of love.** What you see is mostly what you're looking for. Wear love-colored glasses when looking at your partner.

9. **Prevent stress buildup.** Exercise, meditate, pray, play, and breathe. Don't let stress be your default response to life or to your partner.

10. **Clean your emotional attic.** Identify old stuff from your past that is still causing pain or anger. Heal and release it. Get help if you need to.

LEVEL THREE LOVE: CAKE AND ICING

If God is love, and if the creation of the universe was guided by God, regardless of the methods/process used or how long it took, then love is the motivation and power that brought all things, including you and me, into being. It follows that love is the supreme experience we can attain on this earth. I believe that whether we know it or not, our lives are entirely founded on this high state of consciousness I call love.

How can you bring more of this loving consciousness into your close relationships? As with most things, Level Three love begins with you. You will always attract from others more of what is already inside you. When you choose to be in love with life, and when you are able to love yourself in the ways suggested in Corinthians, you are setting up the conditions necessary for attracting a deeply satisfying love relationship—for what my friend Father Bob Spitzer would call, "a sacred partnership."

A happy, relaxed, sacred partnership should be the frosting on the cake of an already happy life. Yet in too many relationships, you ignore the cake to chase after the frosting. In time, you come to realize that frosting alone isn't nearly as satisfying as you'd hoped. In fact, it may come to have a decidedly unpleasant taste. What are you left with? No cake, yucky icing, and a bad aftertaste.

The great thing about sacred partnership is that you get to have it all—a delicious cake (all the things you love about your own life) *and* yummy icing (a supportive mate with whom to share it). The purpose of love is not to complete, rescue or enlighten you. It is not to achieve or sustain the emotional highs of being "in love," either. The purpose of love is to help us become better at loving—loving life, loving ourselves, loving others, and loving God.

SIX STEPS TO SACRED PARTNERSHIP

1. **Commit.** A sacred partnership requires commitment to the quality of the relationship over time, to your own growth and development as a human being, and to the well-being of your partner. Commitment requires patience, persistence and determination.

2. **Connect.** Do whatever it takes to stay closely connected to your partner on all levels—body, mind, heart and soul. Make staying connected an outlet for your creativity and a daily exercise in doing what works.

3. **Communicate.** In a sacred partnership, you strive to identify your own desires and needs, express them respectfully and directly, and listen attentively—with ears and heart—to what's not being said as well as what is.

4. **Reflect.** Think before choosing a course of action or saying something that may wound. Reflect on the past in order to create a more loving present and to help your partner avoid old patterns and pitfalls. This sort of help is always given best in lighthearted and nonjudgmental ways.

5. **Be honest and kind.** Honesty without kindness is brutal. Kindness without honestly is phony. Practice both, together. Learn the wisdom and selflessness of letting little things go, balance giving and receiving, and honor your partner with your full attention and most heartfelt passion.

6. **Grow your consciousness.** The goal of being awake, present and aware in each moment, is shared by all spiritual seekers. Sacred partnership challenges you to spend more of your life in that state of awareness, 100 percent present with your partner, with spirit, and with all that is.

THE SPIRIT OF ENTELECHY
NURTURING SPIRIT IN CHILDREN

Raising Children with a Healthy Self-Esteem

Bringing children into the world may be "doing what comes naturally," but that's only the beginning. The rest is far more complicated. Raising children to have the virtues most of us consider paramount—honesty, integrity, compassion, kindness, accountability, and resiliency—demands a great deal of time and attention. It also pushes us to grow in ways we may never have imagined. Perhaps the greatest opportunity most of us will ever have to improve our own character comes to us through the daily blood, sweat and tears of struggling to be good parents.

Principle Nine is devoted entirely to building your own self-esteem, but young children must rely on us to help them develop a positive self-concept. Behavior is driven by self-image, so it's no surprise that kids with a healthy self-esteem generally act in ways that show it. These children are far more likely to:

- Assume responsibility

- Take pride in their accomplishments

- Act independently

- Rebound from setbacks and tolerate frustration

- Accept new challenges and attempt to learn new skills

- Feel and express appropriate emotions

- Offer to help others

On the other hand, children with low self-esteem tend to:

- Avoid trying new things

- Feel unloved or unwanted

- Disparage their own talents and abilities

- Blame others for their shortcomings

- Feel, or pretend to feel, emotionally indifferent

- Be unable to tolerate a normal level of frustration

- Be easily influenced by others

More than anyone else, it is parents who promote or chip away at a child's self-esteem. Usually, it happens unconsciously. Parents speak without realizing what an enormous impact their words and actions have on how their children feel and behave. Remind yourself to stay aware, monitor your own behavior, and:

Praise effort, achievement and character. Parents are quick to notice and criticize "wrong" behavior, but often fail to give equal time to what's right. Be generous with praise. In particular, use descriptive praise, which specifically identifies the behavior or quality you want to reinforce. For example, if your child finishes a task or chore, you might say, "Your room looks great! You found a place for everything and made it look so nice and neat!" To encourage a talent, say something like, "I really like that song you played. You have lots of musical talent." Don't be afraid to praise in front of family or friends, and praise positive character traits as well as performance. For instance, "You are a very kind person." Or, "I like the way you keep trying even when it's hard." You can also praise children for something they didn't do, such as, "I like that you didn't lose your temper when I said no." Finally, never withhold praise because results are less than perfect. Kids generally have a long learning curve. Praise effort.

Teach positive self-talk. What we think determines how we feel, and how we feel determines how we behave. Teach your children to be positive about how they "talk to themselves." The best way to do this is by example. Next best is putting words in their mouths, as gently and lightly as possible, such as, "I'll bet if you keep trying, you can figure out that problem," or "We lost, but we tried our best, and we can't win them all," or "It feels good to help people, even if they don't always notice right away or say thanks."

Teach good decision-making. Children make decisions all the time but often are not aware that they are doing so. There are a number of ways parents can help children improve their ability to make wise decisions. Help your child to:

1. **Understand the situation.** Ask questions about what he thinks and feels, likes/doesn't like, and wants to accomplish.

2. **Brainstorm solutions.** There are usually several possible solutions or choices. If the child can't see any or more than one, point this out and suggest a few alternatives.

3. **Choose a solution.** Do this only after considering possible consequences. "If you do this, what do you think will happen? How would you feel about that?"

4. **Evaluate results.** How did it work out? Why? What could have been better? Reviewing results helps kids make better decisions next time.

Discipline wisely. Sometimes it is appropriate or necessary to criticize a child's behavior. However, it's the *behavior* that should be criticized, and not the child as a person. *Never ridicule or shame a child.* Discipline should be about teaching, and not punishing. All kids need to learn to accept responsibility for their behavior, and gradually they will become self-disciplined. Toward that end, parents would be wise to see themselves as coaches/teachers, and should aim for discipline that is fair, firm and friendly.

Discipline should always be age-appropriate. Be clear about what you don't like, and what you want to have happen. Keep the tone firm but friendly. For instance, you might say, "When you spill and don't clean it up right away, it makes a mess and is harder to clean up later. Please clean up spills as soon as they happen," rather than "You're such a slob! Why should I have to clean up after you all the time?"

A Dozen Ways to Nurture Spirit in Children

1. **Put parenting first**. Good parents don't think they know it all. They educate themselves about raising kids and have a vision for themselves as parents. They make developing their children's character their top priority.

2. **Check your calendar.** How much time do you spend with your children? *Quality* time can't be planned. It happens spontaneously as a result of an appropriate *quantity* of time together. Make your kids part of your social life.

3. **Teach by example.** All of us learn primarily through imitating what we see. You can't avoid being an example to your children, for better or worse. Being a good example is your most important job. Never stop growing.

4. **Pay attention to what your kids do, watch, and read.** Books, movies, songs, TV, the Internet—all continually deliver messages to children. Parents must oversee and screen the ideas and images that influence their children.

5. **Watch your language.** Words matter. Talk to your kids as respectfully as you would any adult whom you hold in high esteem. Never swear at them or around them. Don't use language that is bigoted, biased or crude.

6. **Be clear about limits and consequences.** All children and teens need limits, which they will inevitably ignore on occasion. Consequences for violations should be promptly forthcoming, consistent and appropriate to the infraction.

7. **Learn to listen.** How often do you tune out your kids? One of the best things you can do for them is hear what they have to say. Don't pretend. Put the newspaper or remote down, establish eye contact, and listen attentively.

8. **Get involved at school.** School is the main event in a kid's life. The nature of their school experiences will influence the course of their lives. Help your kids to become good students and participate in school activities.

9. **Make a big deal of the family meal.** The dinner table is a place where we eat and talk together. It's also where we pass our values along with the mashed potatoes. Eat together as a family, at least once a day.

10. **Help children understand their feelings.** Feelings are a result of the stories we tell ourselves about our experiences, not the experiences themselves. Never blame children for how you feel. Encourage them to identify their feelings—positive and negative—and to express them appropriately.

11. **Encourage options.** When we believe that only one thing or person can satisfy us, we limit ourselves unreasonably. Help your kids see that they can have many friends, many choices, and many activities that bring satisfaction.

12. **Lighten your heart.** Laugh at yourself and with your children. Encourage them to laugh at themselves. The ability to make light of life is an important part of finding joy and contentment, no matter what.

It's a tough world to grow up in these days. Don't underestimate your children. Help them to look for and find a meaningful purpose. Help them to discover the best in themselves and in the world around them. Help them to grow, little by little and year by year, to realize their full potential—in body, in mind, and in spirit.

THE SPIRIT OF ENTELECHY
THE RIPPLE EFFECT

KINDNESS IS CONTAGIOUS

A program called, "Kindness Is Contagious: Catch It," began in a single Kansas City, Missouri public school and has spread to more than 400 schools in the area. Among the activities, the program encourages children to fill up two jars with beans. One jar contains a bean for every time a child receives a put-down, insult, or injury. Another jar contains a bean for every time a child receives a "put-up" or an act of kindness. The purpose, of course, is to increase the put-ups and decrease the put-downs.

A second activity is called, "Pass It On," in which a teacher provides a general overview of what kindness is, and then waits to observe a spontaneous act of kindness among the classmates. When the teacher sees it, she/he gives the kind child an object—a smiley face token or small toy—and tells the child that he or she is now a witness and must pass the object on to someone else who performs a similar act of kindness. The result? Kids *wanted* to be seen performing acts of kindness. They loved it. They didn't care about keeping the token, either.

IT ONLY TAKES ONE SMALL PEBBLE...

...to start those ripples spreading out in the pond, to touch hearts, make a difference, and expand the effects of kindness and goodness on the planet. How does it make you feel when someone smiles and says, "Good morning!" to you as if they really meant it? Or when your arms are full of packages and someone opens a door for you? Or when someone with a cart full of groceries lets you move ahead in line because you only have one or two items?

Early one morning, I was getting a cup of coffee to go at a local Starbucks, when I overheard one of the employees talking about something that had happened there recently. Apparently, someone in the drive-thru had paid for their order, and then added an extra $5.00 to cover the person behind them in line—a stranger who would, of course, never know their name or be able to say thank you.

That stranger turned out to be a woman who seemed quite flustered when the drive-up cashier explained that her coffee had already been paid for by the person in the car that had just pulled away. The woman laughed. She cried a little. Then she did the same thing for the person in the car behind *her*. She paid it forward. And so it went. We don't know how long the chain of giving lasted, but it was long enough to lift the spirits of everyone at Starbucks and everyone within earshot, including, of course, me.

What would happen if everyone on earth made a point of sharing just one act of kindness every day? The world just might be transformed. What if everyone did the same thing as that wonderful book/movie suggested, and "paid it forward?" I'm not talking about some grandiose gesture or anything that takes a lot of your time and energy—although you may be motivated to give it more time and energy, just because it feels so good to do good!

One night, Darcy and I went out to dinner in Beverly Hills, California. At the restaurant, we noticed a well-known actor. We had enjoyed his movies and his talent. We were big fans. He was there with his wife and another couple. We did not want to bother his party. We told our server that we would like to buy him and his guest a bottle of wine. We gave the server the following instruction: "Please tell him thank you and that we enjoy his work and that he makes us laugh." We instructed the server that under no conditions did we want the actor to know who sent them the wine. We did not want to meet him, but just wanted to tell him thanks for his talent.

With these thoughts in mind, are you willing to accept a challenge? Call it your Entelechy Experiment. For the next thirty days, make it a point to share an act of kindness with someone every day. Here's a list of ideas to inspire you.

KINDNESS AT HOME

- Ask each family member to choose someone who has made a positive difference in his/her life. Write thank you notes and mail them together.

- Work as a family to mow and clean up the yard of a neighbor who is frail, ill, or recovering from surgery.

- Clean up litter on a road near your house or in your neighborhood.

- Surprise a family member with breakfast in bed. (My daughter, Devynn, loves this one!)

- When you're out of town, ask a friend to drop off a home-cooked meal for your spouse. Pay it back with the same service.

- When one person is away for a while, arrange a conference call that includes the entire family.

- Ask every family member for three inspiring quotations. Paste them into a book and give it to a grandparent on their birthday.

- On "big" birthday years—sixteen, twenty-one, thirty, forty, fifty, etc.—instruct family members to put their heads together to make a "Great things about you" list and give it to the birthday boy or girl, no matter what their age.

- Surprise your spouse or child with an appreciative note or funny cartoon in their lunchbox, newspaper or magazine.

- Have family members work together on a monthly "kindness project." Document it with photos and put them in a scrapbook.

- Perform a chore that is normally someone else's job when they are obviously busy or otherwise occupied. Don't announce it. Just do it.

- Wash your spouse's or teenager's car and vacuum the inside. Leave a chocolate "kiss" on the dash.

- Call a spouse, parent or child and say, "Hello, I was just thinking about you and how much I love you."

KINDNESS AT WORK

- Take a big bouquet of flowers to work and give a few to everyone.

- Write a note to the supervisor of someone who has helped you, praising their attitude and actions.

- Start a food drive. Ask for help collecting and delivering it. Send thank you notes to everyone afterward.

- Get to work early and leave a brownie or other goodie on everyone's desk.

- Leave some yummy goodies in a central area anonymously, with a note saying how great the people here are to work with.

- Bring a latte to someone who has been working extra hard lately.

- Write a thank you note to the person who made your day or gave you extra service.

- Never let a kindness done to you pass without recognizing it. A big smile and an appreciative "Thank you so much!" will do just fine.

- Leave enough money on the vending machine so someone can get a bag of chips. Put a sticky note nearby saying, "My treat!" so it's clearly no accident.

- Offer to help someone learn the ropes, share your expertise without being asked, or offer words of support, encouragement or praise to someone who is obviously struggling.

- Gather a group of co-workers and attend a fundraiser for a worthy cause.

Kindness in the Community

- Volunteer. Nothing, not even your money, is more valuable than your time and attention.

- Give blood or plasma.

- Adopt someone living in a nursing home who has no family.

- Leave an anonymous personal thank you note or yummy treat for your letter carrier, newspaper delivery person or anyone who serves you.

- Organize a cleanup in the closest park, beach, or public area.

- Slip a twenty dollar bill to a homeless person or someone who is in obvious financial need. "I think you dropped this," is a good way to deliver it, right before you smile and walk away. Don't wait to be thanked.

- Call your local Boys and Girls Club to see what kind of help they could use.

- Organize a clothing or fundraising drive for a shelter. The fastest growing segment of the homeless population is women with children. Do something to help!

- Organize a school supplies and toy drive for a shelter.

- Return your shopping cart to the proper place after loading your car.

- Shovel your neighbor's driveway or mow their lawn.

- Pay the toll or buy the coffee for the person behind you.

- Get rid of the books you won't read again and give them to a shelter or public library.

- Have a teddy bear drive for your local police department or emergency service.

- Become a fundraiser for a cause you feel passionate about.

- Volunteer. Yes, I know, I said that already, and I'll keep on saying it. You have something to give, no matter who you are or what your circumstances. You have no idea how much you will get back or how far the ripples of kindness you create will reach!

Life is short, but kindness is long. Pay it forward. Pass it on.

The Spirit of Entelechy
What If?

What If It Were Your Mother?

Not long ago, I was a passenger on a direct flight from Madrid, Spain to Los Angeles, trying to psych myself into a good place about spending double-digit hours in the air. I was seated in row 300A (or so it seemed), up against the window, rather than on the aisle, which I prefer. After a week that seemed like a month in Europe, every day was crammed full of business meetings, presentations and client social events, all I wanted was to go home. No, that's not quite right. All I wanted was to *be* home—in my own house, my own bed, and with my own family. Getting there was the part I was resisting. Like many people, I truly hate long flights, and I have had too many of them lately.

I figured I could get through it if I could just sleep. Since I am one of those people who can sleep almost anywhere as long as I'm in a semi-reclining position, I hoped to get at least a few hours shuteye. As I settled in, I noticed for the first time that the person directly in front of me was a very tall man with big shoulders. No doubt he'd be reclining his seat as soon as possible, which would cut into my already limited space, especially if I was awake. I wasn't planning on being awake. I would just recline my own seat and soon I'd be asleep. I could work on my attitude later.

When the plane reached cruising altitude, sure enough, the big guy in front of me put his seat back. Ah, well. Just as I had mashed my so-called pillow into position and started to release my seat back, I heard a sort of sad little grunt behind me. I levered myself around enough to see who was there and whether the grunt had been, as it sounded, one of displeasure at my decision to recline. For just an instant, I couldn't believe my eyes. I thought mom had somehow gotten on the same plane, even though I knew she was in Seattle. The woman had the same build, same hair and style of dress, and same glasses.

Of course, in another instant, I could see that it wasn't my mom. What a relief. I didn't feel like flying for fourteen hours with my mother sitting behind me—she is quite a talker. Besides, who was this other old woman to be displeased with me? I had as much right as the guy in front of me to adjust my seat, and I was dead tired—too bad if I was taking some of her space. Someone had taken mine. It was only fair.

Then I thought, "Wait a minute. What if that woman had been my mother, coming home after an exhausting trip? What if she, too, felt weary and irritable? What if the person in front of her put his seat down, practically right in her lap? What if I could prevent that and make her flight a little easier?" So I raised my seat into the full upright position and craned my neck to look back at her once more. She smiled and said, "Thank you, young man." It has been a long time since anyone called me a *young* man.

As I sat there, it dawned on me that even though the elderly woman behind me wasn't my mother, she was very likely *someone's* mother. Then I thought, "What if we all saw other people in that 'what if it was my mom' light?" We would just naturally treat them as if they were someone we cared about. Aren't we all worth that? Does that woman have to be my mother, a family member, or a friend before I treat her with respect and kindness? Isn't just being who she is enough?

Assuming a personal connection with the people who give you grief—thinking of them as people with problems and parents and children of their own—has a dramatic effect on how you treat them. If I imagine the old woman driving the car in front of me at twenty miles an hour as mom, impatience transforms into sympathy. If someone lets me down, I imagine her or him as my mom and I'm not so quick to pass judgment. "Maybe, there was a good reason. Maybe I need to find out before I jump to conclusions and get mad." This kind of "What if?" thinking helps me remember to behave like the compassionate, patient person I most want to be. Maybe it will help you, too.

What If You Could Be A Hero?

The dictionary says a hero is a person noted for feats of courage and nobility of purpose. It takes courage to build your own character and do the right thing. People who can summon the internal resources to do the right thing, regardless of circumstances, are everyday heroes.

Everyday heroes are people whose courage hasn't necessarily brought them fame, but they don't care about fame. They recognize the risk or sacrifice that may be involved in what they're doing, but they do it anyway. They value not just the life of the person they help, but all life. They don't panic mindlessly or react foolishly. They quiet their emotions so they can respond effectively. They stay in control of themselves and make smart decisions. Everyday heroes are willing to take risks and make sacrifices because of deeply held values. They don't just talk about what's important—they act to achieve a meaningful goal.

Everyday heroes are the people we universally venerate—the firefighters and police officers who put themselves into danger to protect others. Their altruism and courage are arguably heroic. Everyday heroes are also teachers, preachers, bankers, brokers, baristas, veterinarians and volunteers—anyone who goes above and beyond to help someone in need, however that need manifests itself.

One universal quality of true heroes is that they don't see themselves as heroes. In fact, they often become uncomfortable with any public attention for their deeds.

You can measure your own heroism by the greatness of the fears you have overcome and the people you have served wholeheartedly. Think back. What fears have you faced? What risks have you taken? What sacrifices have you made to help someone have a better life? Now think ahead. What could you do tomorrow?

What If Everyone You Encountered Came Away With Feeling Better About Themselves?

Imagine that there is someone in your life who always makes you feel good when you are around her or him, even if it's just a brief encounter. Maybe it's the way their face lights up when they see you. Maybe it's their sense of humor or the way they have of finding something to praise or admire about you—the way you look, your accomplishments or talents, your behavior, or your character. Or maybe it's something else—something not so easy to define. But you almost invariably get a lift from being with them, and you look forward to the time you spend together. It might be the woman who hands you your Egg McMuffin or the guy who mows your lawn. Perhaps it's a co-worker, colleague, family member, mentor, or a friend.

Now imagine that that person is you. What would it do for your relationships to be that kind of person? How would it affect your marriage, your friendships, your family life, your on-the-job acquaintances, and relationships with supervisors and co-workers? What would it do for your self-esteem if it were obvious that people really liked being around you, looked forward to their encounters with you, and were always happy to see you when you showed up again?

It *can* be you, of course. How? Make a goal of it, for starters. Affirm and visualize it. Plan for it. What could you do to make it happen? Could you start by giving everyone with whom you spend time your undivided attention? What about really listening to what they have to say? Could you train yourself to be alert for what you might do for them instead of what they could do for you—to offer words of praise, support, affection or admiration every time you were together?

Will the same behaviors make every single person you encounter feel good? Not likely, although a genuine smile, a quip or a few words of praise are safe bets for just about everyone. You will probably have to tailor your behavior to fit the individual you're with. What makes your teenager feel good, may not please your grandmother, and the thing that makes the room service waiter smile, may not work for your boss. Play it by ear, but play it as well as you possibly can.

Does this mean you will be turning into a people-pleasing doormat? Not a bit. Keep in mind that what you are doing isn't about making people like you. It isn't about you at all, although there is no doubt that you will benefit. Even when someone cuts you off in the checkout line at the store, Get Over It and Get On With It. Even when someone at work gets to you, Get Over It and Get On With It. Even when the neighbor leaves their garbage cans out all week, Get Over It and Get On With It.

It's about making someone's day, or a part of their day, and as a result, making the world a better place. That's how it happens—one person at a time. What if...?

THE SPIRIT OF ENTELECHY
AFFIRMING SPIRIT

The following affirmations were created to help you assimilate the material in Part IV and make it part of your life. Choose the ones you like and adapt them or use as is. Remember to visualize, feel and believe in the truth of the words. Repeat the process often.

- I see the face of my mother (grandfather, God, the divine, humanity—use a word that works for you) in everyone I meet, and I treat them accordingly.

- I am patient and kind to everyone, including myself.

- My daily life is filled with opportunities to make other people's lives easier and happier.

- I feel energized and happy when I forget myself and focus on helping others.

- I control my emotions and express them appropriately and respectfully.

- I am willing to risk or sacrifice for the values I hold most dear.

- I honor and value all life, everywhere.

- I respond quickly when help is needed and do what needs to be done.

- I am courageous and bold in living my life and promoting the common good.

- I love interacting with people and hearing their stories.

- I love putting a smile on people's faces and a glow in their hearts.

- I love to smile, and I am good at making others smile.

- I feel great when I do something good for others.

- I find something interesting or endearing about everyone I talk to.

- The more I think and live on Level Three, the happier I feel.

- My spirit expands when I fill my mind with love, compassion and joy.

RECOMMENDED READING

Self-Esteem

Branden, Nathaniel: *Self-Esteem At Work: how confident people make powerful companies,* San Francisco, Jossey-Bass Publishers, 1998.

The Six Pillars of Self-Esteem, New York, Bantam Books, 1994.

The Power of Self-Esteem, Deerfield Beach, FL, Health Communications, 1992.

The Psychology of Self-Esteem: a revolutionary approach to self-understanding that launched a new era in modern psychology, San Francisco, Jossey-Bass Publishers, 2001.

A Woman's Self-Esteem: stories of struggle, stories of triumph, San Francisco, Jossey-Bass Publishers, 1998.

How to Raise Your Self-Esteem, New York, Bantam Books, 1987.

The Psychology of Romantic Love, Los Angeles, J.P. Tarcher Publishers, 1980

Canfield, Jack: *Self-Esteem and Peak Performance* (audio), Boulder, CO, Career Track Publications, 1989.

OPTIMISM

McGinnis, Alan Loy: *The Power of Optimism,* San Francisco, Harper & Row, 1990.

Seligman, Martin: *Learned Optimism,* New York, A.A. Knopf, 1991.

What You Can Change and What You Can't: the ultimate guide to self-improvement, New York, A.A. Knopf, 1994.

The Optimistic Child, Boston, Houghton-Mifflin, 1995

Authentic Happiness, New York, Free Press (Simon & Schuster), 2002

LEADERSHIP AND ORGANIZATIONAL BEHAVIOR

Arbinger Institute, The: *Leadership and Self-Deception: getting out of the box,* San Francisco, Berrett-Koehler Publishers, 2000.

Baker, Dan; Greenberg, Cathy; Hemingway, Collins: *What Happy Companies Know,* New Jersey, Prentice-Hall, 2006.

Bennis, Warren: *Leaders—Strategies for Taking Charge,* New York, Harper Business, 1997.

Reinventing Leadership: strategies to empower the organization, New York, Morrow, 1995.

Rethinking the Future: rethinking business principles, competition, control and complexity, leadership, markets and the world, London/Sonoma, Nicholas Brealy Publishing, 1997 (Rowan Gibson, editor)

Managing the Dream: reflections on Leadership and change, Cambridge, 2000.

The Future of Leadership: today's top leadership thinkers speak to tomorrow's leaders, San Francisco, Jossey-Bass Publishers, 2001 (Gretchen Sprietzer and Thomas Cummings, editors)

Fritz, Robert: *The Path of Least Resistance for Managers: designing organizations to succeed,* San Francisco, Berrett-Koehler Publishers, 1999

Jaworsky, Joseph: *Synchronicity: the inner path of leadership,* San Francisco, Berrett-Koehler Publishers, 1996.

Kriegel, Robert: *Sacred Cows Make the Best Burgers: paradigm-busting strategies for developing change-ready people and organizations,* New York, Warner Books, 1996.

Loehr, Jim and Schwartz, Tony: *The Power of Full Engagement,* New York, Free Press, 2003.

McCarthy, Patrick and Spector, Robert: *The Nordstrom Way: the inside story of America's #1 customer service company,* New York, J. Wiley & Sons, 1995.

SPIRITUALITY AND LOVE

Borys, Henry James: *The Sacred Fire: love as a spiritual path,* New York, HarperCollins, 1994.

Buscaglia, Leo: *Loving Each Other: the challenge of human relations,* New York, Fawcett Columbine, 1984.

Living, Loving and Learning, New York, Fawcett Columbine, 1983.

Hooks, Bell: *All About Love,* New York, William Morrow & Company, 2000.

Keyes, Ken: *Your Life is a Gift, So Make the Most of It,* Coos Bay, OR, LoveLine Books, 1987.

Spitzer, Fr. Robert J with **Robert A. Bernhoft** and **Camile D. DeBlasi:** *Healing the Culture: a commonsense philosophy of happiness, freedom, and the life issues,* San Francisco, Ignatius Press, 200

Moore, Thomas: *Care of the Soul: a guide for cultivating depth and sacredness in everyday life,* New York, HarperCollins, 1992.

Peck, M. Scott: *The Road Less Traveled: a new psychology of love, traditional values, and spiritual growth,* New York, Simon & Schuster, 1978.

The Road Less Traveled and Beyond: spiritual growth in an age of anxiety, New York, Simon & Schuster, 1997.

Welwood, John: *Love and Awakening: discovering the sacred path of intimate relationship,* New York, HarperCollins, 1996.

HEALTH AND SELF-HEALING

Naparstek, Belleruth: A variety of excellent healing imagery and stress reduction audios, published by Time-Warner Audios, along with research information about effective guided imagery techniques, are available from Naparstek's website at www.healthjourneys.com.

Siegel, Bernie: *Love, Medicine and Miracles: lessons learned about self-healing from a surgeon's experience with exceptional patients,* New York, Perennial Library, 1990.

Peace, Love and Healing: bodymind communication and the path to self-healing, New York, Walker, 1990.

Audio Healing Images: affirming and envisioning yourself as an attractive, whole and unique individual, Santa Monica, Hay House, 1990.

IMAGERY/VISUALIZATION

Denning, Melita: *Practical Guide to Creative Visualization: proven techniques to shape your destiny,* St. Paul, Llewellyn Publishers, 1998.

Gawain, Shakti: *Creative Visualization: use the power of your imagination to create what you want in your life,* San Rafael, CA, New World Library, 1978.

Naparstek, Belleruth: A variety of excellent healing imagery and stress reduction audios, published by Time-Warner Audios, along with research information about effective guided imagery techniques, are available from Naparstek's website at www.healthjourneys.com.

Siegel, Bernie: *Audio Healing Images: affirming and envisioning yourself as an attractive, whole and unique individual,* Santa Monica, Hay House, 1990.

SUCCESS, PERSONAL GROWTH AND DEVELOPMENT

Branden, Nathaniel: *The Art of Living Consciously,* New York, Simon & Schuster, 1997.

Taking Responsibility: self-reliance and the accountable life, New York , Simon & Schuster, 1996.

Fritz, Robert: *The Path of Least Resistance,* Salem, MA, Stillpoint Publishers, 1984.

Russell, Peter: *Waking Up In Time: finding inner peace in times of accelerating change,* Novato, CA, 1992.

Sher, Barbara: *Wishcraft: how to get what you really want,* New York, Viking Press, 1979.

I Could Do Anything if I Only Knew What It Was: how to discover what you really want and how to get it, New York, Delacorte Press, 1994.

It's Only Too Late if You Don't Start Now: New York, Delacorte Press, 1998.

Tye, Joe: *Personal Best: 1001 great ideas for achieving success in your career,* New York, Wiley Publishers, 1997.

Nolen, Roland: *Beyond Performance: what employees need to know to climb the success ladder,* Wheaton, IL, New Perspectives, 1999.

Csikszentmilhlyi, Mihaly: *Flow: the psychology of optimal experience,* New York, Harper, 1990.

SELF-TALK

Budd, Matthew and Rothstein, Larry: *You Are What You Say: a Harvard doctor's six-step proven program for transforming stress through the power of language,* New York, Crown Publishing, 2000.

Helmstetter, Shad: *What to Say When You Talk to Yourself,* Scottsdale, Grindle Press, 1986.

Hewitt, William: *The Art of Self-Talk: formula for success,* St. Paul, Llewellyn Publications, 1993.

ABOUT ENTELECHY™ TRAINING & DEVELOPMENT, LLC

Jim Madrid, CEO and Founder envisioned a company where each associate is committed to attaining the best-in-class research and disseminating that research in a process-based format designed for individual client needs and goals. These scientifically based processes clarify the steps to lead organizations and individuals to unprecedented, record-breaking performance. Entelechy works with senior leaders of organizations like Lexus, Boeing, Paramount Studios, Washington Mutual, to build and sustain a knowledge-based organization conducive to such critical elements as individual and organizational learning, empowerment, and innovation.

Since 1997, Entelechy Training & Development has been leading companies and individuals through transformational change with their training, development and assessment solutions. Centuries ago, Aristotle coined the word *entelechy* to describe *the vital force that urges all living organisms toward growth and self-fulfillment*. And like many timeless truths, our name stands for the foundation through which all Entelechy programs are based.

While education and research is Entelechy's foundation with such notable programs as *The Ten Principles of Entelechy and Leading Transformational Change*, measuring employee engagement and return on investment are integral factors of the Entelechy process. With tools that allow you to measure results and predict the future success of your people, Entelechy makes it possible to hire, promote and involve individuals in new corporate initiatives knowing with certainty which people are most likely to do well, advance, remain loyal and produce results for your company. In essence, Entelechy offers a multi-level approach for the training and development of a company's best asset – its people; assessing, training and development and reassessing. Ultimately leading to a return on investment that is scientifically based and unprecedented in this field.

Headquartered in Mission Viejo, California, Entelechy Training & Development has offices located in Spain and Canada.

Entelechy® is a registered trademark of Entelechy Training & Development, LLC.
Ten Principles of Entelechy® is a registered trademark of Entelechy Training & Development, LLC.

For more information about Jim Madrid and products and services of Entelechy Training & Development, LLC please contact us at:

Entelechy Training & Development
27401 Los Altos, Ste. 390
Mission Viejo, CA. 92691
949.218.5587
www.entelechy.net
info@entelechy.net

Gaku
The Chinese Symbol for Happiness

樂